BARKLEY
A DOG'S JOURNEY

ANGEL CITY PRESS

BARKLEY
A DOG'S JOURNEY

AL MARTINEZ

Al Martinez

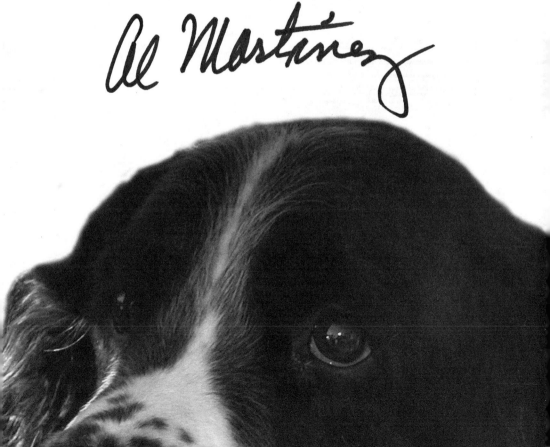

Barkley: A Dog's Journey
Copyright © 2006 by Al Martinez

Designed by Amy Inouye, www.futurestudio.com
California cover map by Art Your World
All photos copyright © Joanne Cinelli

10 9 8 7 6 5 4 3 2 1

ISBN-10 1-883318-60-2 / ISBN-13 978-1-883318-60-4

LIBRARY OF CONGRESS CATALOGING-IN-PUBLICATION DATA

Martínez, Al.
Barkley : a dog's journey / by Al Martínez ; designed by Amy Inouye.
— 1st ed.
p. cm.
Summary: "When Barkley was diagnosed with terminal illness, Al Martínez and his wife Cinelli decided there was no time like the present to spend 24 hours a day and 3000 miles with their wondrous dog. They face not only Barkley's impending end, but come to grips with their own future as they contemplate the roads they traveled" —Provided by publisher.
ISBN-13: 978-1-883318-60-4 (trade paper : alk. paper)
1. Dogs—California—Los Angeles—Anecdotes.   2. Cancer in animals—California—Los Angeles—Anecdotes.   3. Travel with dogs—Anecdotes.   4. Human-animal relationships—Anecdotes.
5. Martínez, Al.   I. Title.
SF426.2.M367 2006
636.752'4--dc22

2006009882

Printed in the United States of America

ANGEL CITY PRESS, INC.
2118 Wilshire Boulevard #880
Santa Monica, California 90403
310.395.9982
www.angelcitypress.com

For Cinelli, who loves all
Living things, even me,
(Most of the time.)

ACKNOWLEDGMENTS

MY GRATITUDE GOES OUT to all who contributed in bringing the story of Barkley into book form and thereby gentling my memory of such a lovely dog. I thank my good friend Chuck Morrell who first suggested it, Paddy Calistro and Scott McAuley for agreeing to publish it, Amy Inouye for designing the final product, and all of the readers of my *Los Angeles Times* columns who laughed when Barkley romped and cried when he died. We all knew him together.

PROLOGUE

ONCE UPON A TIME . . .

Is there any better way to begin a story?

Once upon a time.

Once is where everyone has been, and time is where we are and where we'll be. There can be no greater self-encompassing start to a tale, this tale or any. Especially if it's a journey, and that's what this is. A dog's journey.

Think of travel, and life, as a route to a destination. Think of it as a trip through time. Think of the instances that brighten the journey, flowers along the way, mountains in the distance, trees scraping the lower edges of the sky.

Think of it as moments, the sudden awareness of a single blossom amid massive greenery, the perfume of pine wafting across a country lane, a smile from a stranger, a nuzzle from a dog. Think of it as a game of fetch by a stream fed by autumn rains, rushing over rocks buffed to a dark sheen by years of passage.

I remember these things now in a house grown quiet by a dog's absence. I remember them when I slip behind the driver's wheel of my car to begin a trip, and the back seat is empty. I think of them as I come home and there is no leap to greet me at the door, no nose that pokes into our shopping bags to see if there's something for him.

One wonders at these moments of vacancy how long the feeling of emptiness will last. When will we forget that once there lived a wondrous dog named Barkley who bounced like Tigger, spun like a Santa Ana wind and loved us no matter what we did or how we did it or why. He loved us on the stormiest of days, in the angriest of moods.

How long will it be before my wife and I accept that he is gone and we must, as politicians like to say, move on? Should I at last take down the photographs, and tuck away the memories? At some point, perhaps. But not now. Not as I begin to relive a journey, a life's journey, that wound for almost three thousand miles through the mountains and valleys of California, and along the awesomely beautiful Pacific coast of Oregon, battered by an ocean as old as summer.

There is a story to tell here. Shall we begin?

Once upon a time . . .

CHAPTER ONE

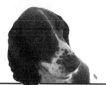

THE JOURNEY BEGAN AT OUR FRONT DOOR.

Barkley bounced into our lives, ears flopping, on a spring day in 1997 and immediately responded to the ringing bell of my fax machine by dashing into my work room and eating the paper the machine was disgorging.

"He's an interesting dog," my wife said, watching him chew and wrestle with the emerging paper, glancing up proudly as he tore into page four. "I hope it's nothing you want." Then she leaned down and hugged him, and I swear to you, he hugged her back. What better way to begin a journey?

Barkley was seven months old. He was born in the

green English countryside and brought to this country by an American woman traveling abroad who had seen him at a farmhouse and had fallen in love with the bouncing English Springer Spaniel. It became apparent to many in the years he graced our house with his presence that he was a universal spirit of endearment in a world grown increasingly cold.

I had written in my column for the *Los Angeles Times* about the death of our old dog Hoover, a stubborn, bad-tempered mutt that no one could ever please and no yard could hold. Among my readers was Suzanne Childs, media director for the L.A. County District Attorney's office. She had brought Barkley from England, but it became quickly apparent to her that, because of a heavy traveling schedule, she couldn't keep him. She was looking for a home and, if we were interested, she would like to see if our environment was adequate. She would not leave her dog just anywhere.

We live in doggie heaven. Our large house borders on twenty thousand acres of state and national park, a wonderland of hills and oak trees, and a view of the distance that stops the heart. It's in Topanga Canyon, one of the last areas of the Santa Monica Mountains with open space still available. The Chumash Indians lived here long ago, and later it belonged to hippies and musicians and those who sought peace from the drums of the city. Writers, artists, actors and others of a liberal nature continue an easy tradition established by prior generations. Horses ride the trails and dogs rule the hillsides.

It was apparent to all of us that Barkley belonged here. Childs let him go with tears in her eyes, handing us his inoculation papers as though she were parting with her firstborn, and we accepted them as though we were adopting an impish child. I've thought many times about that first meeting with the mischievous puppy that began sniffing around our house and standing on his hind legs, front paws on the edge of a table, to see what edibles might be available.

There was something about him that was different from most dogs. Black-and-white with an elegant face and a patrician air, his gaze met other gazes head-on, and his emotions were always apparent. Curiosity shone there and determination and anger and atonement. Chased, he ran. Corrected, he hung his head and averted the glare of his admonisher. He knew instinctively that the house he had come to occupy was his home. He darted through a dog door into his large, fence-enclosed yard as though he expected it to be there, and drank from a large bucket of water as though it was his, putting his whole face and floppy ears into it and dripping his way back through the house.

Then he met Sharmy. If we had planned on owning dogs that were different from one another, we would have planned on Barkley and Sharmy. They were the yin and yang of the canine world, one bouncy and playful, the other already edging into old age, grumpy and unwilling at first to tolerate the habits of a puppy that only wanted to have fun. Sharmy was part wolf and part something else and was known to snap if pressed. Our son had left him with us for a few weeks while he traveled, and then a few more weeks while he thought about building a fence that never got built and then he just became ours by default. In some ways, the two dogs were meant for each other.

We worried at first that Barkley could be hurt by the old grouch that still possessed the strength and temperament to cause damage. But Bark was as quick as a hummingbird, lunging in long enough to nip playfully at the older dog and out again before Sharmy had a chance to respond. When he wasn't sprawled out someplace sleeping, always nearby and in the way, or amusing himself with a toy that squeaked, Bark was after Sharmy, bugging him to play, the way a little brother might torment his big sister, only stopping when he tired of the game.

To say that our new dog adapted quickly as a vital member of the family would be to say that of a new baby who fills a family niche the day he or she comes home from the maternity ward. Before a week had passed, he had adopted an old leather chair with a footstool as his and sprawled out facing our dining room table. When he wasn't curled up directly under Cinelli's feet as we ate, forever eager for a tidbit, he was sprawled out on the chair and footstool, facing us, watching from one eye as we took every bite.

Cinelli was his favorite. He could be found most of the time somewhere near her when we settled after dinner into an evening of reading or watching television. When she left the house he curled up on a mat in front of the door, waiting. When she was ill, he'd settle at the foot of the bed. Like Edgar Allen Poe's cat, his presence added comfort during bad times.

Bark loved children and tolerated their roughhousing with equanimity. When he was very little, our youngest grandson Joshua would attempt to mount him like a horse, throwing a towel over his back for a saddle blanket and trying to hoist himself up on the dog's back. Bark greeted each episode with a kind of weary glance my way, finally just sinking to the floor and sitting to avoid further back-riding attempts. The boy learned to play "tug" with Bark, each taking one end of a rope toy and pulling, until the other gave way. The dog being the stronger could have won every time, but occasionally let Josh win, and then grabbed the end of the rope to start all over again.

His were the most expressive eyes I had seen on any pet we've ever owned. In their depths lay an intelligence that understood the foibles of children, a loving recognition of their vulnerability and their need to play. Those eyes expressed mixed emotions at times, joy and confusion in quick glances. We made contact through his eyes, and although we couldn't teach him to talk (Cinelli tried once or twice), I think he could understand what we were saying.

While he grew in size and intelligence, he never seemed to age in temperament. He was always a kid in many ways. We'd talk to him the way we'd talk to maybe a pre-teenager, explaining, teaching, trying to help him adjust to a new home with new people and new rules. He even understood Sharmy's grumpiness and would edge Joshua away when the boy tried to do to the old dog what he'd do to Bark. That took no training. It was an instinct of the most protective dog I've ever known. He seemed to realize what peril was in a gentle and loving way.

One forgave Barkley his bad habits, even if at the time those habits seemed costly. Cinelli baked three dozen cookies once for a special occasion and left them on a kitchen counter to cool before packaging them for their destination. Barkley had grown quickly over the months and could, by standing on his back legs, reach parts of both the sink and the dining room table and certainly a coffee table where hors d'oeuvres were placed when company was expected. His nose could reach far, and, where his nose failed, an extended paw didn't.

Barkley was an accomplished thief. He stole my cell phone and ran through the house with it, me chasing him and the phone ringing. The ringing was a kind of bugle sound that made it seem as though he was dashing off to war, with me in pursuit, or perhaps bringing up the rear. Cinelli watched us circling the fireplace from the living room to the dining room and around it again to the living room and so, it seemed, ad infinitum. But then he somehow had touched that part of the phone that accepts a call, so that a voice was suddenly emerging from the thing in his mouth and he quickly dropped it. For a moment, he stood looking at it, head cocked, curious, and then trotted away. He wanted nothing to do with a toy that talked.

The cookie theft occurred when Cinelli had left the kitchen for a few moments. When she returned, they were gone, the flat tin of their container empty of every crumb. After standing in the middle of the kitchen wearing a puzzled expression, she asked, "Am I going nuts or did I just bake three dozen cookies?"

"You baked the cookies," I said.

"But they're gone!"

Had she put the cookies back in the oven? No. In the refrigerator? No. In a drawer? No. Had she absent-mindedly thrown them away? Put them in the mailbox? Hung them in the closet? No, no and no. It seemed like a dream, or perhaps a haunting. We've always felt that the spirit of her great aunt, the domineering Margaret Monroe, was loose in our house. We blamed her when anything mysteriously moved from here to there, or sometimes from there to here. But she had never stolen three dozen cookies before.

I was willing to help Cinelli search, but it became apparent after a few moments who the thief was. There was a thumping sound from under the table where Barkley lay in his funny sprawling way, one rear leg somehow tucked under him. The steady thumping was to become a familiar sound as his wagging tail hit the ground in a drumming rhythm. Cinelli and I looked at each other and then at Barkley, whose expression of guilt instantly revealed the fate of the cookies. Never had we seen such a mea culpa on a dog's face. One could almost hear him say, "I did it."

"He ate three dozen oatmeal cookies," Cinelli said, in a tone more of disbelief than anger. "It'll kill him. No one eats three dozen cookies at one sitting."

"He doesn't look like he's dying," I said. "He looks guilty, but, well, content."

"Bad dog," she said, without really meaning it. Mischievous dog, maybe. Or clever dog to have discovered and taken the cookies without leaving so much as a crumb.

"More like ingenious dog," I said. I turned to Barkley. "Bad, ingenious dog!"

We began laughing, and he came out from under the table, almost smiling, somehow aware that he had been forgiven, tuned to the nuances of our moods. The cookies were simply a part of the games he played, like a bouncing ball or a small rabbit toy that squeaked to satisfy the instincts of a hunter, or the nips he took at Sharmy's behind. We loved him for the games as well as for the warmth he brought into our home, adding a dimension to the environment that almost shone. His luminescence was internal, glowing from within.

He seemed to radiate good health, and we would wonder later how his last journey had come upon us so quickly.

CHAPTER TWO

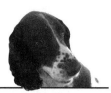

BAD NEWS SEEMS TO HAPPEN AT NIGHT, when misfortune moves on the edge of the darkness and terrible things evade the light. Our bad news came with a phone call at two in the morning. We were in Wales, a peaceful and fiercely independent "colony" on England's western border, where the time is eight hours ahead of L.A. We were asleep when my son, Marty, telephoned us in our hotel room in Swansea, the home of poet Dylan Thomas and of the celebrity-of-the-moment Catherine Zeta-Jones. That very day we had explored the home under construction that would theoretically someday be occupied by Jones and her husband-of-the-moment, Michael Douglas. A guide had taken us to an area of Swansea called the Mumbles to show us the house, and then to a fish restaurant where she occasionally visited while in town. He was as proud of her relationship to Swansea as he was of one of the preeminent poets of the twentieth century.

"Something's wrong with Barkley," Marty said.

The words had the impact of a punch in the stomach. Both Cinelli and I had noticed from time to time that his appetite occasionally lapsed for no reason. Normally, he gulped down his own food, and then tried to eat Sharmy's too. But Sharmy had similarly gulped down his food, so they both left their bowls at the same time to explore the other's for whatever crumbs might remain. If Bark had a little something left and Sharmy wanted it, Bark would give way, less out of fear than generosity, or maybe a respect for age.

As we thought about it later, we would remember there were moments when Bark seemed lethargic, and times when he crawled rather than bounced on the old couch in our bedroom, which we had recovered in leather just for him. Once Cinelli and I had climbed into bed, and only then, he would snuggle down, his head on a pillow, and go to sleep instantly, opening his eyes occasionally to make certain we were still there. I can still see him looking sleepily at me, when I glance over at his empty couch. In the morning, he would remain there until we arose, and then it was up and outside to greet the day.

If it was raining, so much the better. Bark loved rain. It was in the breed, the water dog who'd leap into a stream after ducks shot down by his owner. The only bird he ever got at our house was one he caught in mid-flight, and brought proudly to us. We're not bird killers, but it was too late to save this one. Punishing him for following his instincts would have been like reprimanding a baby for stepping on the cat's tail. We laid the bird to rest and hoped Bark would thereafter leave the creatures alone.

When he did get drenched in the rain or in a small, rubberized pool we bought for him to cool off in L.A.'s often intense summer heat, we'd have to catch him before he leaped through his doggie door into the house and trailed water in every room. Cinelli and I would take turns using bath towels to dry him off, his thick fur retaining enough of the moisture for him to spray the room by shaking it off. He loved taking a bath, too, and would often jump into my bathtub, his bathing place, and wait for someone to come in and add water. A rubber ball left in the tub when he'd finally give up prospects for a bath that day was evidence of his effort. But when we took him to a dog-care facility to have him bathed, he would resist going in the door with the strength of a bull pulling on the other end. If anyone was going to bathe him, it was going to be us, not a stranger. Bark never did learn to accept "outside" baths. It was either us or no one.

The phone call.

It hurts to think about it even now.

"He's not eating anything," my son said, "and he seems barely able to move."

Cinelli had picked up the other phone extension. "It could be because he misses us. Emotions play a big part in the health of a dog so sensitive."

We could sense his sadness when we left the house even for a few hours, and his abounding joy when we returned. But it was different this time.

"I don't think so," Marty said. "I took him to the vet and she's suspicious that he might have something more serious. She wants to do some tests."

"Do whatever's necessary," we both said, almost in unison.

We knew he would. Marty's love of animals, of anything in nature, is deep and abiding, whether they are coyotes, raccoons, possums, deer or even an occasional mountain lion, all of which roam our canyon community. One of the most traumatic moments of his life, at about age eight, was when a dog we called Squirt was killed by a speeding car. We were camping by a lake north of L.A. The car didn't stop or slow down. We found an animal hospital, but it was too late for Squirt. He was Marty's special dog. Still resonating in memory are my son's words, said with sadness and a child's sudden awareness of fate and cruelty, as he looked down at his pet: "He didn't come here to die."

Death is an abstraction in the lives of the young until someone or something close is suddenly gone before old age takes him. Squirt was a package of abundant life that was terminated in an act of cruelty. In Marty's case—and I don't know how this happens—sorrow made him more caring and more aware of the deficiencies that fate can deal out. His sensitivity to Barkley's illness was born of that. He sensed it. He knew.

When we hung up after his call to Wales, there was a long silence in the room. We too sensed that something was indeed terribly wrong with the dog that had been a part of us for eight years. We continued to speculate that his lethargy could be emotional, but we both knew deep in our hearts that it wasn't. Our vet, Holly Scoren, who has tended to the health and welfare of our animals for many years, knew at once that it was something serious, and ordered tests.

The few days that passed had Cinelli and I tense with anxiety. We were thousands of miles away and helpless to take a direct part in Barkley's health. Then the worst news anyone could imagine: our beautiful, gentle, happy little dog had acute lymphocytic leukemia and was given no more than nine months to live.

A pall lay over the few days that remained of our time in Wales. Touring the green hills once trod by the armies of Rome and driving along an oceanfront as rugged and beautiful as any we had ever seen should have been the visual sedatives that calmed the big-city demons that have always been a part of my life. I have been a journalist for half a century, and my clock ticks toward deadlines twenty-four hours a day. As a columnist who covers L.A., just being in the city is work. I can't separate events of the day from the essays they might make. I have to change environments, to retreat into a difference that is the antithesis of a metropolis. Wales was perfect. The countryside is both ancient and pastoral, with castles on the horizon and sheep dotting the green hillsides. Time is grander there, more awesome than the minutes we worship.

When we returned home, Barkley seemed his old self, greeting us at the door with an enthusiasm that was equal to his most excitable moments. To say he leaped into our arms would minimize the reception. He leaped and hugged and then ran up and down the hallways, spinning and barking. He never had an in-between. When he wasn't curled at our feet or sprawled on his chair, he was leaping into the air after a ball and catching it in his teeth. It was his favorite game, played in the gentleness of the evening: bring a ball, have it thrown into the air, catch it and trot a victory lap around the fireplace. His record was five catches in a row, his reward simply the pride of the catch. When Cinelli or I were too busy to play, he'd stand in the middle of the room, ball in his mouth, staring. He was building on our guilty feelings, waiting us out, and he usually won.

"Is there any chance that the diagnosis is wrong?" I asked the veterinary oncologist, Sue Downing, who was treating him. She was a large, gentle woman recommended to us as the best in the business. She shook her head. "None at all," she said. She had already prescribed a series of medications intended to keep his energy up and make him as comfortable as possible. Chemotherapy was recommended. It would be expensive and possibly have side effects. She would control them as the treatment continued. But it wouldn't cure him.

There was no question that we would do what we could for Barkley, despite the expense involved. It ultimately amounted to thousands of dollars. Throughout the course of the treatment, there were ups and downs. When his appetite failed, we looked around for a food that he couldn't resist. That turned out to be pork roast. The finest canned dog foods didn't tempt him, nor did premium ground beef or any of the other goodies we offered, except on occasion. Then at dinner one night, looking at us from his chair, he was sniffing the air and seemed more than casually interested in the pork loin. I gave him a piece. He devoured it.

"Well," Cinelli said, watching him go for it from a dish on the floor, "I guess we've come up with his dinner of choice." He ate every bite and then shoved the dish across the room, licking up what was left. When he was finished, he looked up and almost said, "Any more?" It was a discovery that would sustain Barkley to the very end. Sometimes we bought a pork roast exclusively for him, and sometimes we shared one. His appetite went up and down over the course of his treatments, and his stomach often rebelled at any kind of food after chemo, but in between, he gained weight on pork roast, sometimes with a little toast stirred into the juices. Cinelli prepared his food with the loving care of a favored friend, and Bark was all of that.

When the cancer had been in remission for some weeks, we again asked Dr. Downing if there was any hope at all. She explained once more the inevitability of his destiny. There would be moments of life beyond our wildest expectations, she said, but then the illness would suddenly, and explosively, strike him down. We should love him and enjoy him while we could.

It was during a period when the disease was in remission that we decided on a journey tailored for Barkley, to places that would allow him the freedom to run and explore. He loved to go bye-bye, and responded to the very term by rushing to the door and waiting, trembling with anticipation, his eyes filled with excitement. This, we decided, would be a grand bye-bye. We laid out a month-long course on a map through the mountains and wide valleys of California up to the rugged coast of Oregon. Three thousand miles with Barkley in the back seat.

"It's a big, big bye-bye," I said to him. He bounced to the door and waited.

Let the journey begin.

CHAPTER THREE

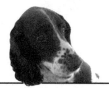

"The only journey is the one within."

—Rainer Maria Rilke

WE TRIED NOT TO THINK OF IT as a last journey for Bark. It was, instead, an adventure, only the second time we have ever taken a dog with us on any kind of a trip. The first was years before when a mutt we called Hoover accompanied us on a cross-country jaunt in a rented camper. Hoover would not be contained, and utilized every opportunity to escape. He did so in the bayous of Louisiana, a friend's house outside of Boston and in Buffalo, New York, just on this side of an international bridge that joined the U.S. with Canada. Like a draft evader of the 1960s, he would have made it into Canada had he kept going. But, unlike the draft evaders—most of them at least—he stopped to urinate against a power pole, thus affording us the opportunity to snap a leash on him.

Barkley displayed no such tendencies to escape. He would run when given the opportunity, but stop and return instantly when we called his name. Unlike Hoover, he harbored no desire to leave us forever, or to lose himself for at least the length of time it took to drive us crazy. Hoover ran for no apparent reason toward no apparent destination. I would have just let the damned fool go, but Cinelli is kinder in her attitude toward animals of limited cognizance, such as fish, turtles, gerbils and Hoover. So we ran after him each time, like children chasing the wind.

⚜

Events tend to blur as one pulses through time and space, leaving a trail of scenes and activities that can be easily forgotten in the quickening pace of today's world. Moments become lost in a jumble of memories that fade one into the other, and eventually sink back into darkness. Years of travel to places like

Africa, China and Russia have taught us to record these trips on film and in journals in order to keep them a part of our lives, before they vanish completely.

I have before me, as I write, photographs taken on the Barkley trip, and a page open to a journal that begins "Day One. Lone Pine." I envision Barkley sprawled out on the back seat of our Camry on a bed of blankets especially prepared for him by Cinelli, laid over a sheet of plastic, just in case. It was his home on the road and he loved it. In the trunk was stored a large, collapsible doggie "cage" with a thick mattress, his room each night in our motel. Next to the cage, an icebox that contained, among other things, cooked pork roast.

Lone Pine is about two hundred miles northwest of Los Angeles, and was a first stop at the outset of our journey. One skirts the lower edges of Death Valley to get there, past vast expanses of sand that end in distant mountains, and past dilapidated shacks, roofs collapsed and doors swung open, that were the abandoned dreams of those who sought peace and solitude in the isolated landscape.

A town of sixteen hundred souls and one traffic signal, Lone Pine boasts that it is the gateway to Mt. Whitney, at 14,494 feet the tallest peak in California. It is also the home of the annual Lone Pine Film Festival, featuring cowboy shoot-'em-ups that were once the weekend matinee diversions for kids like me. Because of its variable terrain, old westerns were made there over the years, with actors like Hoot Gibson, Tom Mix and Gene Autry. In later years, recognizing its almost eerie moonscape, filmmakers turned it into another planet for *Star Trek* movies and into eerie dreamscapes for episodes of *The Twilight Zone*.

Temperatures rose along the desert's rim, and Cinelli worried about Barkley's comfort. The car's air conditioning was on, but she decided that he also needed the window cracked slightly open so that, his nose poked out, he could sniff the distance. The problem was, it let the hot air in and defeated the air conditioning.

"You worry more about the dog than you did about our kids," I said teasingly as she held a water dish for Bark.

Her response was quick: "The kids didn't lie in the back seat with their tongues hanging out, panting."

It was the kind of logic that defied debate. For all the years we had motored with our three children when they were young, not once had I seen them with their tongues hanging out, panting. Our kids and Barkley all loved the open road, the idea of going somewhere. One wondered what was going through his head as the scenes flashed by like a cinematic panorama of mountains and desert, and as he barked or growled at an unseen nemesis along the lanes heading north.

"I wonder if he knows it could be his last trip," Cinelli said one evening, as we drove. She turned to Bark in the back seat. "This trip is just for you." He offered a smile, but it was a guarded smile, as if to say, "Sure, but the last trips I took I was prodded, stuck with needles and given stuff that tasted bad. Why should I trust you now?"

We reached Lone Pine in the late afternoon and were prepared to hassle motel owners to allow Bark into their rooms, assuring them that he would spend the night in his cage, and that we'd clean up any unlikely messes that he made. California is noted for its pet-friendly accommodations, and not one turned us away, although a few either charged extra or asked for a refundable deposit. On the first night, we were charged three dollars more for a room so ratty that whatever Bark might have done to it would have probably improved it. Assured of at least a place to stay, we sought out a restaurant called Seasons, the only good sit-down eatery in what seemed like hundreds of miles of fast-food stands. Because we decided never to leave Bark alone in a motel while we dined, he was in the back seat of the car parked outside of Seasons. We had requested and waited for a window booth, so that we could see him and he could see us all the time we were in the restaurant, and hear him as he barked at those who, out of arrogance or ignorance, dared to pass by. I don't remember what we ate, but I remember that we ordered pork loin to go, hold the salad, the mashed potatoes and the cauliflower. A little bread, however, would be nice.

In addition to his cage, Barkley's equipment also included a length-adjusting leash with a flashlight attached, and a pooper-scooper with a plastic bag for disposing of the dog's "leavings," for lack of a more genteel word. We took turns walking Bark, and I found it not the most agreeable of tasks. There is something vaguely humiliating standing there, looking the other way and pretending you're not involved with it, while the animal defecates. Even more demeaning is the necessity to scoop it into the plastic container to throw away. Sometimes, in areas specified for such usage, one came in contact with others awaiting their pet's need to, well, poo-poo, creating moments of the strangest kinds of conversation one is likely to engage in. Somehow, discussions of anything involving beauty, such as sunsets or flowers, seem inappropriate under the circumstances. I would prefer silence in such cases, but since we are likely to share a common chore, at least a mention of the weather or "Hey, how about them Dodgers!" seems necessary.

Out of Lone Pine on a day as bright as heaven, sailing north along Highway 395, paralleling a mountain chain that will grow into the mighty Sierra Nevadas. We're traveling up the eastern spine of California on a road that rises and dips like a roller coaster ride, through terrain that offers chalky-white peaks in the distance, and small settlements that cluster along the route. We pass Manzanar, where Japanese Americans were interred during the Second World War in a violation of their civil liberties that we have only recently come to face. This is not new territory to us, but a common destination for many long weekends out of L.A. in a century-old hotel we have frequented in the town of Independence, down the street from a French restaurant of adequate, if not spectacular, fare.

We are wanderers, Cinelli and I, and have sought far horizons through most of our lives, increasing the mileage to far-flung continents as funds became available. Even in our seventies, as time collapses behind us and shortens before us, we are planning trips to India and to the Amazon and beyond, eager to taste the sweetness of new wonders and to tingle with the anticipation of new adventures. I will admit that Cinelli tingles more than I tingle, due to a greater willingness to poke into the unknown, but I am ultimately with her wherever her instinct takes us. "Make the sign of the cross," as my mother used to say, "and get on with it."

It was all new to Barkley who, when he wasn't napping, acknowledged the newness with sudden barks. This could be startling if he happened to have his nose over my right shoulder as I drove, which was occasionally the case. I had the feeling at such times that he was listening to our conversation and would have joined in had nature given him that ability. It was just as well, however, that he couldn't communicate in a humanly manner. The likelihood was, he would have sided with Cinelli in any kind of domestic argument, and I would have been at a loss to counter them both. As it was, we shared some musical preferences played either on the radio or on CDs. He seemed to listen to those he liked, generally jazz or classical, especially the arias of Maria Callas, while turning away from country-western or rock.

But even if music is the voice of heaven, there were times when Bark just didn't want to hear any of it, whatever its source. When a dog wants silence, a dog wants silence. I tried getting him to sing along with me, but he would have none of it. "Good taste," Cinelli said. "He's a solo act."

We rolled out of Lone Pine singing "Tumbling Tumbleweeds," convinced that the journey was going to work. Barkley ignored us.

CHAPTER FOUR

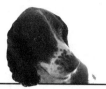

THE ROAD TO MARKLEEVILLE snaked precipitously upward in curves that looked down thousands of feet to the valley floor in appropriately named Alpine County. There were no guardrails on the way up, and it occurred to me that I was risking my life, not to mention Cinelli's and Barkley's, in order to reach a town of sixty-five permanent residents at 5,501 feet. Even the dog seemed puzzled, but not my wife. We were in the Sierra Nevada Mountains, and she was fascinated by scenes that evolved as the afternoon lengthened: distant peaks that vanished into fading shades of blue, and the colors of autumn burning into the slopes of a cloudless day.

"It's gorgeous," Cinelli said, "look quick!"

It was the emotional equivalent of asking that couple in the movie *Open Water*, a man-and-wife scuba diving team accidentally abandoned at sea, to admire the ocean scenery while they were under attack by great white sharks.

I looked when I could in quick glances as I drove, then finally stopped at her insistence to stare in wonder at the gold, coral and amber leaves of the aspen trees, set afire by streaks of sunlight and shimmering with an intensity of color in an ambient breeze. At such moments, one comes to realize how surrounded we are with beauty. Look upward, look outward, past the wars and the anger, past ancient hostilities, to the glow that endures even as we wonder if humanity will survive the millennium. Spring renews, repeating each year a story of resurrection rooted in nature's annual surge; and autumn, a gentle pause between seasons, reminds us that even though winter is coming, wonder lies ahead.

I walked Barkley as Cinelli took pictures of the autumn leaves and talked to him about what I was seeing in the season's luminescence, and about what lay ahead for him, and for all of us. Dying is not the best thing we do, but I have faced it in war, in a cardiologist's hands, on the street and while wracked with the convulsive high fevers of blood poisoning. On the night before open-heart surgery, I walked to a place on a hillside behind our home, where the view is westward toward the Pacific, and came to grips with the possibility that I could die. I'm not usually metaphysical in my approach to death, but I could foresee at that moment a walk among the stars when the life force finally weakened and faded; I could envision an energy flowing like silver ribbons through space, gleaming in the darkness, a glory beyond which anyone could imagine even in the fussy confines of temples or cathedrals.

I talked to Bark about life's uncertainties because I knew his life was limited. But then again, I'd say, isn't the life span of every living thing limited? Every tree and mountain and river and ocean? I'd point out that there's evidence, bits of fossilized sea life, that even a part of our canyon was an arm of the Pacific a millennium ago, an ocean that has since receded into time. The era of dinosaurs was limited, and who knows how long suns and moons and planets and planetary systems survive?

How much of all that philosophizing Bark could even begin to understand is problematic, but I suspect by the way he stood silently and looked directly into my face as I spoke, that he might have gotten some of it. I liked to think it eased the realization of what he faced. Even during the times he lay on the floor of the veterinarian's room receiving chemotherapy and doses of medication intended to bolster his strength and lessen the side effects of the chemo, he appeared to look deep into my eyes, and I wondered then, as I wonder today, if he was trying to read my thoughts, and to understand where real truth lay, when words failed. I have a photograph of him at just such a moment that somehow says it all.

❦

Markleeville is the kind of town one passes through without even noticing it was there. Founded in 1861 by Jacob Marklee, who was later shot dead in a land dispute, it consisted of one motel, one gas station and one public telephone in a small cluster of life that also included a general store, stocked mostly with supplies for fishing and hunting, the Wolf Creek Restaurant and the Cutthroat Saloon. Barkley loved it. He ran barking through an open field bordered by towering pine and fir trees, the sentinels of the mountains, and growling toward the red-barked manzanitas that thickened the underbrush.

When I informed Sandy Matlock, the owner of the motel called the J. Marklee Toll Station, that the key to the room we were renting didn't work, she replied that it didn't matter, there wasn't any crime in Markleeville. Living in Los Angeles, I was naturally suspicious of a town without crime, peril being an important facet of the urban culture. She assured me, however, if assurance is the proper term, that bears lumbered out of the woods occasionally looking for food. One trashed a small coffee shop that is part of the motel, another wandered into the saloon during the mountain equivalent of the happy hour.

"All the drinkers fell off their bar stools," a waitress informed me later, serving up a steak so massive it covered the plate (half for me, half for Barkley). "I still don't know whether it was the beer or the bear that knocked 'em down." Her laughter was a cougar's screech, trailing behind as she strode toward the kitchen, tray held high.

I asked Sandy why she had left a home in L.A., where she was raised, for the remoteness of Markleeville. She replied, "A bad marriage." I didn't pursue the conversation, and she didn't offer more. But I could understand how the peace of isolation might beckon. Loneliness is relative to contentment. One can be lonely in a crowd and happy in isolation. I figured she just ran from whatever memories might still have been plaguing her, leaving them behind in the noisy streets of L.A., and emerging whole in the thin air.

But as I thought about it later in a discussion with Barkley, you can't really escape from your past. Running away from a bad situation is like trying to get away from yourself. Memory follows like a wolf in pursuit of prey, always just behind the runner in the shadows of his yesterdays, padding along on silent feet. Bark always seemed to be thinking about what I was saying, but since he hadn't yet mastered human speech, I had to interpret his thoughts. I could imagine comments like, "That makes sense to me" or "I'm going to sleep on that" or "A lot of damned nonsense."

No sound broke the stillness of the icy night we spent in Markleeville. A feeling of the coming winter was in the air, a pungent aroma of champagne and spices, the distant presence of a new season waiting at the edges of the forest. Stars never seen in the city filled the sky, so vast and bright in the absolute darkness that one could almost comprehend infinity. Barkley gloried in the night. He barked at the intrusive presence of the moon and sniffed the vaporous smells of the wildlife. If a bear should have come into town, he'd have greeted it, tail wagging, while the beast stood on its hind legs and stared in confusion. Our friendly little dog knew no enemies and feared no danger. Every living entity was his friend. We could learn from that.

I suspect that we could have brought Bark into dinner

with us, so casual were the arrangements in what had once been a hotel fueled by the money from gold and silver mined in the nearby hills and streams. Now fishermen in hip-high boots dine there, and off-road vehicles bearing hunters prowl the forests during the right seasons. But while the French regularly bring their dogs into their cafés and bistros, it just isn't the custom in America, so Bark sat behind the wheel of our car parked, just as in Lone Pine, on the other side of a window where we had dinner, saving him half a steak. While he traveled in a back seat especially prepared for his comfort, it was behind the wheel for him when he was in the car alone, waiting. I suspected that with the slightest encouragement, he'd have been on my lap as we traveled the high roads.

My lap was a favorite spot in his puppyhood, and I welcomed him there as I read or watched television. He couldn't read, I'm sorry to say, but I think he could pick up on some of the shows I had on. Occasionally he'd lose interest and turn away, just about the time that I was losing interest and turning away. His presence on my lap wasn't my usual form of acceptance. I'm not the kind of guy who normally cuddles puppies. But as I've said from the beginning, Bark was different. We were joined at the mind, a single unit of emotion and instinct. He was different. As he grew to be a sixty-pounder, he'd settle at my feet, his chin resting on my footstool, his gaze fixed on me, wondering. Wondering *what*? I can only guess.

As I sit staring out a window of my home in Topanga Canyon, watching the new spring leaves of the oak trees rustle shades of emerald into the sun, I visualize Bark sitting patiently at the wheel of our Camry, contemplating the route life would take him. I see him suddenly glance to the left and to the right in the quick movement of a sentry on duty, a gesture he seems to have adopted only for this motor trip. I superimpose a photograph of him on my desk over the images his memory evokes, and the picture is complete, the pieces drawn together, a matrix of eager and abundant life that exists no longer. I turn from the window and I sigh deeply, wishing that I could cry.

We left Markleeville late the next morning, long after the fishermen had risen to seek their streams and the hunters their prey. I do neither as a pastime and am uneasy with the killing of animals. But we found ourselves reluctant to leave, for fear that, like the mythical village called Brigadoon, it would vanish into the night, not to appear for another hundred years.

While no singers or dancers graced this small and rustic village, it remains in afterthought the quiet kind of place that one seeks in terrible times. As I write, the blood of terrorism's innocent victims flows in the subways of London and in the neighborhoods of Baghdad, as the rate of killing increases in Iraq. The world tumbles downward in free fall, and the future seems to rest in the bombers of a planet that trembles with despair. One needs a quiet corner at such times, and one needs a dog.

CHAPTER FIVE

THE WORLD MEETS AT THE REST STOPS OF CALIFORNIA. More than one hundred million people visit them every year, and the number increases as tourists from around the globe target the Golden State as their destination; and the way to see it best is either on foot or from a motor vehicle. Since very few would take on the formidable task of walking seven hundred seventy miles from Mexico to Oregon, an intricate system of highways and freeways are the routes of choice. The rest stops have awaited the wanderers in one form or another for one hundred fifty years.

Barkley spotted the one he wanted before I even

noticed it in a clump of trees off Highway 395, the main north-south route on the eastern edge of the state. He barked his insistence to pull over.

"I can't believe he knows about rest stops," I said, parking next to a van that seemed filled with multiple families. They disembarked one at a time, both kids and adults, like a scene from an old Marx Brothers movie, where an endless stream of unlikely characters emerge from a single phone booth.

"He's one smart dog," I added, counting a total of sixteen van-riders.

"He's more than a dog," Cinelli replied.

She saw his IQ as slightly higher than the average politician's, and just a little lower than that of a Ph.D. in Euclidean geometry. There were times, she once informed me, that she preferred the dog's company to mine, pointing out that he was non-argumentative, always listened to what she was saying and didn't drink martinis.

The van I was watching wasn't a big vehicle, not one of those oversized buses used to haul around old ladies or churchgoers. Watching its riders stretch and work out the kinks, I wondered how they all had fit inside. They had to be carefully stacked. Another automotive miracle on the long and lonely road.

Unlike many European rest stops, California's offer neither restaurant nor gasoline station. They're usually clustered in trees and are equipped with bathrooms, state maps on large boards, vending machine food and soft drinks, picnic tables and areas to walk dogs.

"It isn't just dogs they walk," an attendant said as I hooked an expanding leash on Barkley. It was equipped with a stop button and a flashlight to both control his enthusiasm by allowing varying lengths of line and to be able to see where we were going when we dog-walked after dark.

"You mean like cats?" Cinelli asked.

"I mean like turtles and rabbits and even fish."

"They walk fish on a leash?" She asked it straight-faced.

I could have mentioned the northern snakehead, an air-breathing fish that, well, walks or crawls or wriggles from pond to pond and screws up an ecosystem by eating the local fish. But I didn't. There was no doubt she was putting him on, which she is able to do with amazing dexterity.

The attendant observed her with incredulity.

"You can't *walk* a fish!" he said. "They walk the bowls that the fish are in!"

"Yes. Of course," she said, still expressionless.

Barkley was becoming restless just standing there and I saw no point in adding to the conversation, although the idea of walking a turtle, or even a rabbit, was more than just a little intriguing.

As it turned out, there was a cat-walker among us, and Bark took more than just a passing interest in its presence. The Springer Spaniel is a hunting dog whose pedigree goes back to the mid-1800s in Spain, where he was used to flush birds from their cover. Splashing through streams was a part of the dog's job, which would explain Bark's attraction to water, any water, whether he was being bathed, running through the shower of a garden hose or drinking by sticking his entire head in a bucket and emerging dripping from nose to neck.

What I couldn't determine was why he stole paper from wastebaskets and off the dining room table where Cinelli often did her bill-paying work. It is one thing to find used Kleenex under a chair, quite another to have to search the house for a missing check. All we could pray for was that he hadn't eaten or mangled it so badly that it couldn't be cashed. As he grew, he stopped jerking paper from my fax machine, but still stole paper off the table whenever he could. I discovered on an Internet website that stealing toilet paper off the roll was one of the breed's traits. Barkley, a dog of infinitely good taste, did not, thank God, indulge in that type of border-line scatology.

"He steals to gain our attention," Cinelli said.

"He gets mine."

"Exactly."

They are, as I've mentioned, hunting dogs, and the presence of a cat, leashed or not, excited his instincts to pursue. Unless you have been dragged along by an unusually strong animal with unlimited stamina you have not experienced the pain of having your arm jerked from its socket while trying to hang on to a leash. One moment only curious, the next he was streaking toward the cat, leaping forward with the speed of a racing car that goes from zero to sixty in no seconds at all. Even illness failed to overcome his compelling instincts at that moment. No cat ought to go unchased when a dog is around.

We had two cats at home, Cat One and Cat Two, identical twins eventually done in by the coyotes, and while Barkley often observed them with interest, he never attacked. The cats, however, apparently understood his instincts, and chose to look down on him from the safety of the roof or a tree limb, just in case. But the feline at the rest stop, walked on a leash by a pleasantly fat lady, was a cat that did not rate the protection of familiarity. To Bark, it was just game and he went after her like a ground-to-cat missile. Cinelli shouted and he stopped, but not before sending a wildly panicked feline halfway up a tree, strangling from the sudden tightness of the collar around its neck.

We apologized profusely to the lady and admonished Barkley, who hung his head and looked up in abject dismay, for either having been scolded or not catching the cat; we couldn't tell which. The woman and her husband were from Topeka, Kansas, where you had to buy liquor in state stores, which were often closed. Both happy-hour drinkers, they were more than pleased to be able to buy booze in California just about any time they wanted wherever they were. While that might not be the most attractive asset of the Golden State, I guess it's one. My only experience in Topeka was to interview a preacher who assured me that all of the sinners in America eventually ended up in Los Angeles. Granted, I've come across a few in the basin, but I have also found a surplus of sinners in Washington, D.C. It is, in fact, a veritable anthill of sinners.

I thought about that as the couple from Topeka drove away and as Bark pulled me along through the rest stop, glancing back occasionally to see if I were still attached to the other end of the leash. Is there any domestic creature freer of sin than a dog? None of a dog's actions, even those we might question, are premeditated, but are either driven by instinct or breeding. I would never have a pit bull in my home and don't understand those who do, unless they're drug dealers protecting a safe house. While it may not be true across the board, the pit bull is by breed a fighter, and its inherent nature is to attack. That makes him dangerous. Many are the news stories of them savaging owners, neighbors and passers-by with often deadly effect. Had Barkley done in the Topeka cat, it may have been manslaughter, or catslaughter, I guess, but not murder.

We made it out of the rest stop without further trauma. Bark made friends with every dog there, male and female. "You think he may be bisexual?" I asked Cinelli. "I think you may be bipolar," she replied. Dogs don't have the same cultural hangups possessed by humans. They go around smelling each other's behinds without any feelings of guilt or embarrassment. Barkley used to take it a step further by greeting women guests to the house by putting his nose into their crotch as they entered through the front door. This naturally startled some of the more staid among them, but people in the canyon where I live are known for their liberal, free-spirited, animal-understanding attitudes and just pushed him away, unbothered by his display of trans-species affection.

We noticed as we prepared to head out that Bark had a little more trouble than usual hopping into the car. He'd start up and then pause momentarily before half clawing his way into the back seat. Cinelli and I exchanged glances as he instantly settled into a sleeping position, but we said nothing. Nothing needed to be said. The exhaustion of his illness was creeping into his life.

Northward.

Greenville, Susanville, Burney, Dead Horse Summit, Weed. The names seem to belong in a cowboy-country travel guide, not in a state known more for its sophistication than its wranglers. Look beyond L.A., San Francisco and San Diego, despite their luminous reputations, to find the real California. Small towns dot the vast northern mountains, the rich valleys and the southern deserts. Whiskeytown, Death Valley, Angels Camp, Jamestown, Grass Valley. California is gold country, cattle country, silver country, agricultural country and wine country. And it's also John Steinbeck country in the fields and around the old fish canneries of Salinas Valley where he worked and met the characters that adorn his flawless prose.

It was becoming increasingly icy as winter nudged at the edges of fall. The air rang with the clarity of wind chimes, and smelled of rosemary and pine. We were grateful for extra blankets in Greenville, where we stayed in a complex of cabins among ancient oaks. The desk clerk was an anomaly in a region of outdoor purity, chain-smoking in a small, cluttered office, wincing against the smoke that curled up from her cigarette. A basset hound at her feet eyed us suspiciously as we checked in. Barkley waited in the car, barking for us to return.

Moving from place to place and climate to climate seemed to both attract and confuse Bark. It gave him new places to explore and new things to bark at, but I suspect that he missed a sense of place, a familiar territory that animals like to establish. It wasn't home; it was a lot of different homes that one had to adapt to, where everything smelled different. I tried once by sniffing side-by-side with him to smell what he was smelling, to identify the differences in a new location, but it was beyond my capacity. Cinelli found us sniffing the air together and worried that I might start marking my turf by urinating on surrounding shrubbery. I assured her that I had no such intentions.

Greenville was a town of two thousand souls, one saloon and no restaurant. Because of a well-stocked market, Barkley dined on pork loin, while we ate in a pizza parlor/ hamburger stand that had stopped selling burgers at 7:30 when they ran out of meat. The front page of the *Indian Valley Record* featured a half-page photo of the Greenville High homecoming queen, and the story of a woman who had her and her dog's hair dyed in matching shades of lavender. It was that kind of town.

It rained the next morning, drenching the grounds of the compound. Barkley jumped and spun in the rain, barking as he leaped toward the weather, a dog's dance in autumn. I can't count the number of times he stood in the rain and got himself soaked back in L.A., while Sharmy curled up in a corner of their mutual dog house and remained perfectly dry, looking up occasionally to observe Barkley's peculiar behavior. It took Cinelli half an hour, two bath towels and a hair dryer to make sure the dampness was gone.

"Why in God's name does he just stand there and get soaked?" I'd ask, and she'd say, with affection, "Because he's Barkley."

Her feelings for the loving little dog were not based on conditions, but on an acceptance that was all embracing. His habits needed no explanation. They were Barkley. That was good enough for her.

We left Greenville in its soft rain and drove through Susanville with its unremarkable ambience, where once I had covered a fight between a teacher and a preacher over the booking of a blue movie at the town's only theater. We would return to it later on the way home, trying to take comfort in a poetic admonition to "focus on the journey, not the destination."

Both the moment and the journey belonged to Barkley, and we were sharing it with him. So we treasured the moment and drove through time's pleasure.

CHAPTER SIX

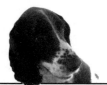

ONCE UPON A TIME there was this perfect little town called Etna. It's still there actually on the west side of the state in the Klamath Mountains, but there's such a picturesque quality to it that it seems almost like a movie set that will be dismantled and packed away when the film is completed. It's a combination of Mayberry and Cabot Cove, whose realities existed only on film, the quintessential small town of schoolhouse, ice cream parlor, red brick church, homemade peach pie and a concert in the park.

I had chosen Etna for the trip because it had been selected by *Outside* magazine as one of America's dream towns, and coming from a metropolis where few are happy and practically no one content, I wanted to be in a place that is completely at ease with itself. Many, if not all, of its 781 inhabitants described it in glowing superlatives, and even those who leave seem to return. It's about as typical as a place gets. One expected to see Opie riding his bike down Main Street, past Nona's Nook, on his way to cookies and milk with Aunt Bea. At about four thousand feet, Etna has been a well-kept secret.

There was a twilight concert in progress in a park across the way as we rolled into town. A rockabilly band was twanging it up to the delight of a couple of good old boys in the motel room next to ours who sat on a universal porch, drinking beer, smoking cigarettes and amusing Bark by spitting out into the field, a pastime that I found unsavory but which Bark thoroughly enjoyed. It's a form of entertainment I never would have thought of. They'd spit and the dog would chase it, barking, and they'd laugh like hell. One wonders how the cowboys might have amused themselves when a dog wasn't around.

Getting there was almost as much fun as being there. An early snow had dusted Mt. Shasta and its surrounding peaks, visible through the high country on ribbons of road that we often had all to ourselves. They dipped and rose in well-regulated rhythms, affording us flashes of snowy summits telescoped through rows of pine and fir that lined the two-lane highways. It was almost as though the roads had been built to focus on Shasta, which rose with mighty insistence on the horizon. Despite the growing chill of the weather, Cinelli insisted on leaving the windows cracked so Bark could savor the perfumes of the mountains that floated out from the surrounding forests. His welfare was always on her mind.

Angling toward the coast from the east side of the state, we crossed I-5, a north-south high-speed freeway through the heart of California, in the late afternoon and reached Etna an hour or so before twilight. Like Markleeville, it's a stopover for hunters and fishermen, and also for rock climbers, kayak boaters, hikers and others who enjoy sweat-based sports. There was only one motel in town, a tidy, one-story strip of twelve units by a grassy field and a creek, which Barkley instantly claimed as his own. He raced through the open spaces and jumped in the creek as though God had put them there for his pleasure. I had the feeling that he was filling his life as much as possible with the natural beauties that Earth provided, to remember as he trotted off for the last time. He would stand for long moments staring at a stream as though absorbing it, the way we might study a particularly glorious sunset streaked across an ocean's horizon, trying to isolate it forever in a corner of our memory.

There's not a lot of entertainment in Etna. The teenagers, for instance, seem to congregate around an ice cream parlor called Dotty's, which in itself was an edifice out of Mayberry. They hang out under an oak tree totally unaware that down in the big cities their counterparts are banging it up at rave parties, where ear-splitting noise, marijuana and a dangerous turn-on drug called Ecstasy are combining to fry the brains of a whole generation. I'm not saying that the only alternative to a teenage orgy is spitting and barking, but it sure amused Barkley and his new best friends.

In so many ways, dogs don't require a vast amount of choices to keep them happy. In the San Fernando Valley, and elsewhere in L.A., there's a park specifically for dogs, where you can remove their leashes and let them run and meet with other dogs. To Bark, it's a kind of Disneyland without the high prices. He seemed to know we were taking him there the minute we started up Laurel Canyon from the Ventura Freeway. In addition to his eager eyes, his jaw would hang open and he'd start panting with anticipation. When I removed his leash at the park, he exploded with the heady new freedom, dashing into dogdom's realm and making friends instantly. That field near the motel provided the same kind of running room, but without other dogs.

I asked the Etna motel owner, a laconic, slow-talkin' man named Bart Jenkins, why the motel was so full midweek. He shrugged and said, "Dunno." He was in a closet-sized laundry room folding freshly washed towels. He and his wife Pam moved out of Yreka (population 7,313) to get away from big cities and, as he put it in a sparsity of words, "No motel here. Built one." They did a lot of the work of washing and vacuuming themselves. When I asked what he thought of Etna being chosen as one of America's great places, he replied, "It's a nice little town, I guess." I wondered briefly if, in his emotional lexicon, that was high praise, but then he went on to mention somberly that there'd been one homicide last year, "First one in a long time." He didn't say what it was about, but one could imagine a fatal fight over the ownership of a doily.

When twilight turned to night, the band across the way turned exclusively to rock, which sent Bark's friends to bed. "It's not so good now," one of them remarked, spitting. The sound bounced around under the heavily forested hills of the Klamath Mountains, where bears and cougars lived, and occasionally came down out of the mountains to bug the humans. I'm not crazy about bears, even the cute ones that wander out of the San Gabriel Mountains bordering L.A. and make themselves at home in hot tubs and in the shade of sub-urban trees. I don't live far from Malibu, the home of the unfortunate grizzly bear lover Timothy Treadwell, whose adoration was requited in Alaska, where he and a girlfriend were killed by the animals they were attempting to befriend. That's the very reason I have never attempted to curry favor from anything likely to eat me.

The band played under a large, open-sided blue tarp tent, and the small crowd that gathered sat at picnic tables. As a chill set in, the band was left mostly alone, but it kept rockin' away like it was playing Carnegie Hall.

I took Bark to hear the music and he quickly became the center of attention. In Mayberry, I guess everyone knows when there's a new dog in town. He made the rounds like a politician running for office, greeting everyone and accepting their pats and pets with a smile. I mean, he actually did smile. He was with people. It was his kind of environment, but he was receiving more attention than the band, so we didn't stay too long, which seemed to disappoint those he attracted. There's a showbiz saying that cautions actors to avoid being on stage with dogs or children, because they become the focus of an audience's attention. In Bark's case, that's certainly true.

We dined that night, although "dined" might not be

the right word, at Bob's Ranch House restaurant, where farm hands who didn't need menus because they ate there every night gathered to enjoy the house specialties of chicken and rice, and beefsteak stuffed with cheese and hot chili. I had the beefsteak, and it wasn't too bad, although I doubt if you'd find it in New York's Café des Artistes, where Bill and Hillary dine, or at L.A.'s Bastide, a restaurant so exclusive that there's no name out front. Just an old English "B." There were racks of fishing poles on the wall at the Ranch House and a lot of talk about hunting dogs and shotguns. One man put down a newspaper long enough to remark to the only waitress in the place, "Lots of problems in L.A." To which, ambling on by, she replied, "Never been there, never wanna go."

Bark waited patiently in the car just outside our window, knowing he'd have a special meal later. He did. Meat loaf, which he ate with such gusto that we wished we had a portable freezer with us and could buy a few pounds to take on the road. Bark's appetite had become iffy. Even pork roast didn't always appeal to him. It was yet one more indication of leukemia's terrible inroads. Another was the crying sounds he'd sometimes make in his sleep, prompting Cinelli to rise and comfort him as she would a baby. But then they'd pass, and at dawn it was our old Barkley again, as though night had somehow refreshed him, and the new day had urged him into its buttery sunlight.

We finished dinner with homemade peach pie. Homemade was the operative word around Bob's Ranch House. One might even guess that Bob himself did most of the cooking, but I didn't ask. I dropped Cinelli off at the motel and Bark and I toured the town. I let him sit in the front seat, which he loved to do. There's not a lot of traffic in Etna. You could walk down the middle of Collier Way, which is the main street, from one end of town to the other and never get run down. Try that in the City of Angels and you wouldn't go three steps before the polished chrome front bumper of a low-riding, flame-streaked Chevy would send you flipping through the smog like a stunt man in a *Matrix* movie.

We drove up and down the side streets, Bark and I, past a well-kept school, homes that dated back to the early part of the twentieth century, Martin's Gift Shop, the Scott Valley Bank, Don Murphy's Pharmacy, the Main Street Garage (there was actually a Main Street but it was only a side street), a hardware store, a perfect little brick church and, well, a lot of other picturesque places. Etna is proud of what it is, and doesn't intend to change a thing. To hell with the politicians and environmentalists and anyone else who might want to reconstitute the city in a different image. Small towns that know what they are don't need dogma-oriented social "specialists" telling them what they've been doing wrong for a hundred years of mountain survival. That's a little like telling Lance Armstrong he's been pedaling his bike wrong at the Tour de France.

In the 1940s, a move began in Etna to create a new state called Jefferson, which would have included parts of Northern California and Southern Oregon. Locals in both states decided they didn't like what was going on in the capitals of Sacramento and Salem. The move was heating up when World War II came along, shifting everyone's priorities, but it hasn't been forgotten in Etna, where the *Pioneer Press* bills itself as "the state of Jefferson's official newspaper." An Etna grandma who, in gingham dress and flat-heeled shoes, truly fits the role of a country elder, loathed the *damnedenvironmentalists* because they wouldn't let her shoot mountain lions that might be endangering the kids in town, including her grandchildren. She left no doubt, though, that if she did happen to see a cougar slinking down Collier, she'd be coming the other way armed with a 12-gauge shotgun.

Bark and I bonded on our long, slow ride through a darkening town. I'd reach over and touch him every once in awhile, as though to affirm his living presence. The length of his illness allowed time to consider its consequence, and while it provided space for a kind of loving sadness, it also offered room to appreciate what we had. Glancing at him sitting next to me in the car, eyes bright with the anticipation of a new experience, of seeing something or smelling something that he had never sensed before, created a feeling in me I can't explain. Call it a sudden realization of destiny or, as Ralph Waldo Emerson put it, a moment that vibrated "to some stroke of the imagination."

I parked for a while and let Bark run. The perfect camouflage of his black-and-white fur let him disappear into the shadows that formed at the edge of town, where the forest truly began. I could see his shape in the moonlight and flashes of the white stripe on his head, and then nothing, as he ventured cautiously into the woods. I called and he returned at once, as I knew he would, because dogs understand better than some humans that home is where affection lives, and to wander from it is to experience unknown perils. Soldiers find comfort from battle at home, and sailors find safety from the sea. One is sustained by the warmth and permanence of home's enclosures, and unfulfilled if they don't exist. The term "homeless" describes more than a person without a place to live, but a state of being that transcends any physical abode. Loss is an element of vagrancy. Sorrow accompanies those who wander the streets.

Letting Bark zip around in the dark probably wasn't a great idea, but he wasn't all that crazy about a leash, so I gave him his freedom now and again. A leash impeded him. His strength was such that he could drag you through a forest if he was determined enough, or get all four legs entangled in the damned thing in his roaming forward, backward and in circles. Some dogs might get one leg entangled and then step out of it, but Barkley could very easily get so tied up he could hardly move. Forced to stop, he'd just lie on the ground and wait for Cinelli or me to free him so he could do it again. I tried to explain the proper arrangement of a leash and his legs, but he never really got it. Funny old dog.

When it was time to return to the motel, he jumped into the back seat of the car then, remembering, into the front seat, because that was his privilege this cold and golden night. I think back on it with such pleasure, combining the mountain perfume and the mountain chill with the perfect silence that embraced us. Barkley had a home and he knew it. We had Barkley, and we shared our home and our lives with him. "You're a good dog," I said as we pulled up to the motel. He jumped out, ran into the center of the adjacent field, looked up and barked at the moon. It was his bark of appreciation. I almost felt like barking back.

CHAPTER SEVEN

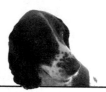

THERE ARE ROUGHLY FIFTY-THREE MILLION DOGS in the United States, and I'm sure that most of them live in Topanga, the Santa Monica Mountains community that Cinelli and I have called home for the past thirty-two years. This is doggy heaven, where God's little roamers, both mutt and pedigree, enjoy a degree of freedom unlike any other community in the Los Angeles basin. There aren't any breeds of dangerous dogs among them, as far as I know. No pit bulls or Rottweilers, but barky, waggy-tailed canines that, even fenced in, are happy to see you go by.

Other than dashing up and down our loooong driveway

like a leopard chasing a dik-dik and going for some arm-pulling walks, Barkley was content to spend time in the house and in his own large private yard. He considered his area of interest, however, to extend at least a mile in every direction, and anyone within that radius got himself a warning to stay clear. If he were in the house and sensed an intruder (a hiker or a tricycle rider or an old lady with a walker) within his defense perimeter, Bark would leap through the dog door like a circus animal clearing a ring of fire and sound out his warning. But then if you approached him, he'd love you to death. The warning was all show. He was just doing his job, protecting what was his.

A dog, by the way, can hear sounds two hundred fifty yards away, while the human hearing range is about twenty-five yards. So even if you tiptoed and whispered, old Bark would know you were coming. His presence in the house was always a comfort and generally less expensive than the high-tech security systems in homes protected by electronic bells and whistles. His keen watchdog abilities were a special comfort to Cinelli when I had to go out of town on assignment and she was alone in the house. He seemed to know the difference between someone on the front porch and a squirrel on the roof, reacting to one with a bark and to the other with a yawn. We noticed that on rare occasions he would take a growling dislike to certain visitors, a plumber maybe or a washing machine repairman, and we'd always wonder what Bark knew about them that we didn't.

Canis familiaris has been man's best friend, and woman's too, for about twelve thousand years. His heritage goes back to a small, weasel-like mammal called Miaci that existed sixty million years ago, plus an eon or two. From Miaci came Tomarctus fifteen million years later, who was considered to be the progenitor of dogs, wolves and foxes, not counting Barkley, of course, who was a breed all his own.

You get interested in stuff like that when you have a dog that is unlike any dog you've ever had. My first dog back in East Oakland was a mutt named Buster. He'd been clipped by a car, which damaged a hind leg, so he skipped when he walked, which made him the most unusual dog on 64th Avenue. While he may have looked the part of a happy dancer as he bopped along, Buster was essentially an ill-natured animal that enjoyed chasing anyone around and was known to nip a bit when he was within range. He was a small dog with far less than a bulldog's jaw power so he didn't even break the skin. In his later years, he stopped chasing, but hung around all of us kids and glared at everyone. Cinelli feels that a lot of my personality is rooted in Buster's early influence.

There is some credence to speculation that dogs tend to pick up their owner's traits over a period of time and that humans tend to choose dogs that resemble them in some ways. I'm not exactly offering this as proof of the theory, but there's a big, bulky kind of guy in our canyon who walks his dog almost every morning. The dog is a St. Bernard. I watch them occasionally as they pass our house and have noticed that they do somewhat look alike, both being kind of slow and heavy and maybe a little dull. I will say, however, while the dog drools a good deal, as St. Bernards do, the man doesn't.

Barkley had a mercurial personality that seemed to reflect my own, which is probably why we connected. I won't say he was exactly moody, as I tend to be, but even before he became ill, he did have a tendency to want to be alone occasionally. Perhaps, at such times, he was pondering a problem relating to his life. More likely, he was simply doing as I do, which is staring into space and daydreaming his way into heroic images of himself: the first dog on Mars maybe or the dog that jumped to the controls of a 747 when the cockpit crew passed out and piloted it to a safe landing. A canine version of Walter Mitty.

Dogs have enjoyed a good deal of notice throughout their history, including a place in the stars where Canis Major,

the great dog, follows his master, Orion, as he makes his annual journey through the sky. There's also Sirius, the dog star,
which is thought to cause the dog days of summer, that time of
year when the whole world slows down. The Greeks mytholo-
gized dogs, especially Cerberus, the three-headed dog that
guarded the gates of Hades. The Romans adopted dogs both as
pets and as fighters in their Coliseum, while the ancient
Hebrew and Muslim cultures found them unclean, which, as we
all know, they can be. On the other hand, certain breeds like
the greyhound enjoyed royal treatment in England, where their
ownership was restricted to kings. Others had to work for a living. Small dogs called Tipsters were used to run on treadmills
that turned the spits over great open fireplaces. Cinelli was
pretty sure Bark would have never done that kind of work.

"Any dog whose favorite sleeping position is on his
back with all four legs in the air doesn't strike me as a laborer,"
she said one day, glancing at him taking a mid-day nap in his
feet-up position.

In more recent times, dogs have taken their places in
the public realm by means of television and the silver screen. It
all began with Rin Tin Tin, who made the first of twenty-two
movies in 1925, and escalated from there. Next came, in no
special order, Asta, Lassie, Toto, Snoopy, Goofy (a sort of man/

dog), Sandy (who immortalized "arf"), Benji, Beethoven, Murray, Moose, Lakia (the space dog), all those damned Dalmatians (101 to be exact, pursued by Cruella De Vil) and a whole bunch of others.

I associated mostly with Asta, the dog of Nick and Nora Charles in the *Thin Man* movie series. We both enjoyed our martinis dry, and it didn't matter back then whether they were shaken or stirred or served in a glass or a bowl. While Asta has gone on to his reward, I still sip a dry one occasionally in his honor. Well, actually, in anyone's or no one's honor, but never out of a bowl.

Barkley was a handsome dog whose princely bearing attracted attention. Among those who noticed was a friend who happened to be a film and TV producer. He was at the house one day and wondered if Bark could take commands. I sensed that it was a seminal moment upon which the future often turns. Unfortunately, at the time, Bark was asleep on his back, legs in the air, which was not his most handsome pose. Alerted, however, he stood, shook himself awake, and looked every bit the movie star dog that he could be. But then:

"Is he trained at all?" the producer wondered.

"A little. But he's very smart and quite cooperative," I assured the man.

"Okay then," he said, "let's have a look."

I called the dog, patting my lap in a friendly manner, which normally had him bouncing across the room and in my face. Not this time. He stood looking at me.

"Here, boy, c'mon, Bark, come to papa."

He didn't move.

The look on his face said nothing. He just didn't *feel* like coming to papa or to anyone else at the moment.

"Barkley," I said, growing tense, "come *here*, boy."

No response. It was like he was frozen. One wonders at such times what goes through a dog's mind? Was he asserting his independence, or did he understand quite well what was going on and wanted nothing to do with show biz? I spent twenty years writing for television off and on and can't say that I blame him, but I still wouldn't have minded sharing in some dog-engendered income.

I met an animal psychic once who swore she could read a dog's mind, and in fact could communicate with the animal psychically. I asked her to send a mental message to her dog, one of those large drooling beasts that witless people keep in small apartments, to come to me. She stared hard at him, eyes focused, jaw set, veins bulging in her neck, for about five minutes. The dog finally got up and went into the other room.

"He hasn't been sleeping well," she explained. I understood. My psychic capacity is always lowered when I suffer from insomnia.

Back at our house, the producer was patient but less intense than the psychic.

"Maybe he's just nervous," he said, trying to be kind.

I could imagine Barkley as Lassie, streaking through forests and across open fields to bark frantically for attention from his owner in their humble, but clean and well-kept, farm house.

"It's Timmy," the man says, interpreting the wild barking for his simple, but steady, and also well-kept, wife. He listens to the barking. "Timmy has fallen into an open well, south of town, near the old Rockner Place"—listening as Bark gives directions—"just across from Farley's barn, where old man Kramer used to live before his wife, a sinful woman named Emma, left him for the town drunk!" And off they all run . . . except for Barkley, who is lying down, exhausted. "Let's get Timmy!" the man shouts back. "Please, Barkley, hurry, we must save our boy!" Barkley rolls over on his back, legs up. Fade out.

The producer rose and said, "Well, I guess I'd better be going. Thanks for lunch, and"—patting Barkley—"see you later, boy." I could sense the amusement in his voice at a dog that wouldn't perform, even on the brink of stardom. When the man was gone, Barkley almost instantly wagged his tail, barked at the door, chased his toy rabbit, leaped on my lap and looked into my face, smiling and eager.

"You're too late," I said. "Someone else got the part."

Not that Barkley wasn't trainable. We hired a professional once to begin his training when Bark was just a puppy. He was smarter than most dogs and picked up on the commands right away. When he chose to respond, he did so instantly. But when he was otherwise occupied or simply not in the mood to follow orders, he could be absolutely inert. Bark always knew just what he wanted. For instance, he slept at night on a small couch that we had recovered in leather especially for him. It was his couch, and his alone, only a few feet from our bed, and if someone accidentally put anything on it other than the pillow upon which he rested his head, he would stand and glare at the object and wait until it was removed before he jumped up and settled down, even though there was sufficient room for him too.

If, however, he didn't choose at the moment to go to bed, nothing could get him to climb the stairs. He knew what "Bedtime, Barkley!" meant and, in the right frame of mind, would bound up the stairs, wait at the top until we joined him, then leap onto his couch and almost instantly fall asleep, head on a pillow, oblivious to the movement around him. Although I will say if it was a different kind of noise outside the house, the watchdog in him would trigger the kind of deep-throated barks that would frighten an army away and startle us into a heart-pounding state of alertness.

But, not in the mood, he would linger at the bottom of the stairs despite orders to come to bed, defying me with every expression on his face. He was dead weight when he wanted to be, and I wasn't about to carry him up two flights of stairs to our bedroom and tuck him in. Leaving him alone downstairs was not an option. He could open cupboards and certain drawers with his nose and was inclined to eat whatever he found: packages of rice, raw pasta, bread, fruit, cheese, crackers . . . you name it.

"This is a dog," Cinelli used to say, "who will one day run for Congress." Then on to the presidency. We could do worse.

CHAPTER EIGHT

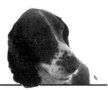

FLORENCE IS A PRISTINE LITTLE TOWN on the Oregon coast, with ocean-gray inns and rows of antique stores, and the ghost of an exploding whale floating through it. Tourists visit by the thousands each summer to marvel at the beauty of waves crashing over the rocky shoreline, churning vanilla foam onto the land and spraying the air with Tiffany diamonds. Only a few of the tourists come because of the ghostly presence of the whale. It blew up long ago and the memory is fading. The rest are just wanderers to the sea, riding bulky campers into town, pulling trailers or cramming themselves and their belongings into and atop dusty automobiles.

Barkley's primary interest in being there was the freedom to race across the white sand like a sun sprite in pursuit of the wind. Many who go there, dog or human, have been emotionally uplifted by the tidal currents of the Pacific's endless surges and retreats, isolated from stress, detached from the land that binds them to their daily lives. Barkley enjoyed that same feeling by his proximity to the ocean, barking at the waves, puffing from the exertion, electrified to high-voltage animation by the exhilaration of the sea.

We drove to Florence to visit old friends, journalists who had trod the same paths I had in the early years of my newspapering career. Gayle Montgomery worked with me at the *Oakland Tribune*, covering politics in the tumultuous 1960s as the Bay Area went wild from Berkeley to Palo Alto in a whole variety of social movements and riots. He retired and moved to Florence some years later, glad to be in a clime of fewer screams and sirens that comprise the shrill concertos of the big cities. Sal Veder was a Pulitzer Prize-winning photographer for the Associated Press who joined us covering the daily campus wars, and later became a part of our drinking and poker clubs. He was visiting when we came by, accompanied by an old Golden Lab called Sophie. Barkley was in heaven.

Both men took instantly to him, but why not? He

vibrated friendliness from every part of his body, trembling with anticipation when a stranger entered the room, taking quick, small jumps in his or her direction, eagerly shifting his position backward and forward as a gesture of his desire to be a pal. It was a dog's equivalent of greeting the world with a smile and open arms. Bark loved everyone, except maybe cats and small rodents. There were no rodents in Florence, but Gayle had two old cats, Mr. Baker and Maxwell. They stayed pretty clear of the dogs, looking down at them from the safety of a fence-top, taunting them with stares and occasionally meows, the way cats do.

Before coyotes got them, Cat One and Cat Two were the wariest creatures I have ever known, including a lot of paranoid writers in my social group. Getting the cats into the safety of a back utility room for the night was an exercise in frustration I do not intend to repeat. Getting the writers in would have been a lot easier. A martini and a pork chop and they're there.

The cats would stand in the doorway when called, listening and staring, refusing to take the steps that would bring them into the room itself and away from night-hunting predators. I would coax, I would purr my love for them, I would promise them their favorite food, I would do everything but fall to my knees and beg them to come in. Well, actually, I guess I did that too. I never knew why they would suddenly agree it was safe to enter and shoot in. On one occasion, after about thirty futile minutes of trying to lure them to their food, I finally said, "To hell with you!" and shut the door just as Cat One had decided to enter. The closing door caught his neck, which caused him to yowl more in surprise than pain and run like the Hound of the Baskervilles was after him. Fortunately, I hadn't *slammed* the door or I'd have been humming a dirge for him right there, and L.A.'s animal activists would have been climbing in my window, but it rapped him enough to send him reeling into the night. Neither cat came in for a month, and then only after hours of assuring them I was only trying to feed them, not do them in.

At Montgomery's place, Sophie, of undetermined age, apparently didn't see too well and spent a lot of time barking at the metal cat figures on the fence. Bark, on the other hand, knew exactly where the cats were and would have gladly brought one home for dinner, like a hunter with a duck in his teeth. Even ailing, his leap was phenomenal, and I worried about Mr. Baker and Maxwell. They were twelve and fourteen years of age respectively and never could have dodged Barkley had he decided to leap after them.

As it was, Bark had a great time with Sophie, yapping and bouncing around like a puppy. His last test before we left for our journey showed his cancer in remission. The oncologist said it would go that way. There'd be good days and bad days. And then it would hit him with sudden and paralyzing impact, and Bark's romp through life would be over. But when he was feeling okay, it was like old times. His energy level was high and his bounce like that of a gazelle flying across the Masai Mara.

He was never hostile to other dogs, even when bigger animals on leashes went at him, challenging every effort of the leash-holder to keep them under control. While other dogs, thus under attack, might jump at the chance to do in an attacker reined in by a leash, Bark would just stand there, not cowering but not hostile, still hoping that the other dog's anger would fade and they could still be friends, like a boxer out of his league praying for détente instead of a brawl. He even tried smiling at them, but they usually kept up their aggressiveness until their owners tugged them away with sheepish apologies. Bark may not have been a fighter, but he feared nothing. I imagine that, if forced, he would have done okay in fight.

The exploding whale, meanwhile, had assumed mythological heights, like a unicorn or a dragon, but it was real enough. Newcomers to Florence had heard about it, but a lot of them were willing to dismiss it as urban legend. Old timers who knew it was true often preferred not to talk about it all. They wanted Florence to be known as something other than a town soaked in stinking whale guts and blubber.

It happened in the winter of 1970 when an eight-ton gray whale beached itself and died on the gleaming sands of Florence, just south of the small, tidy downtown section. Crowds gathered at first, but then backed off when the smell of the rotting forty-five-foot-long behemoth became overwhelming. Something had to be done. The state was called in and then the Navy. There is no better way to make a bad thing worse than by calling in the federal government. After deciding not to bury the carcass because it might be dug up by dogs or souvenir hunters, the two bureaucracies agreed to blow it up.

Their belief was that a half-ton of dynamite would blast the whale into confetti and it would just disappear. Wrong. A television reporter who covered the event said it looked like "a mighty burst of tomato juice." Blood, guts and blubber rained down upon the beach, the highway and the surrounding homes. One huge chunk smashed in the roof of a new car parked nearby. "We were," the reporter wrote, "in a massive blubber shower."

Even today, a year after Barkley's last journey, I keep

wondering what he'd have done under certain circumstances. Would the beached whale have teased his interest or would he have considered it just so much debris on the beach, like driftwood or clumps of seaweed to sniff at? I doubt that, had they buried the carcass, he would have tried to dig anything up. Bark wasn't a digger, for bones or anything else, as far as I knew. Hoover, Bark's predecessor, dug endlessly under the dog yard fence, like a prisoner of war looking for a way out. He often found it. But Barkley was always content with his surroundings, inside and out, and hardly ever pressed to run free beyond the confines of our acre-plus yard. He had his own hill to rule and his rush to its top seemed a constant journey, a burst of vitality that was the explosive equivalent of fireworks.

If we suspected at all in his early years that anything was wrong with him, it was when he seemed to almost stop in mid-bounce, when his energy was abruptly cut off, as though a switch had been suddenly thrown. Cinelli and I can recall times when we wondered about Bark's health even in his puppy stage, when his legs seemed to suddenly give way or when his appetite, normally characterized by eagerness, disappeared. We wondered at his puppy-like awkwardness that saw him flatten out occasionally when rushing down the stairs, but ascribed it to the floppiness of his youth. Mostly he was a dog filled with life, eager to play, anxious to run, straining at the leashes that confined a soul afire with the exhilaration of being. The inner dog was up and running.

The importance of dogs as companions, guards, guides and helpers has been acknowledged for ages, even back to their supposed use in ancient societies to ferret out vampires and zombies. Studies have been made of their behavior and of their impact on modern cultures. How we react to them is supposed to determine how a people react to each other. But how dogs matter emotionally on an individual level is beyond an ability to categorize. I discovered this during a moment in the Korean War, and it has haunted me ever since.

It occurred in the summer of 1951 when our Marine regiment was in reserve. We'd talked a big, awkward, loping sort of guy named Fred to submit to hypnotism as a form of entertainment. A hospital corpsman was the hypnotist. Fred was one of life's victims, a loner, no relatives, no mail and few friends. He went under easily and as a post-hypnotic suggestion the corpsman gave him what he said was a candy-striped dog, one that he loved beyond anything he had ever known.

When the corpsman brought him out of it, Fred awoke cuddling the invisible dog, talking to it with a gentleness he had never revealed. At first, it was a big laugh, but when someone tried to take the dog from him, Fred sent him sprawling with a punch to the face. An officer demanded that the fun and games end, at which point, Fred ducked into his tent, still clutching the imaginary pup, and emerged with a loaded .45. No one was going to touch his dog. It was all he had. It was all he might ever have.

More than that .45 sobered the moment. We realized what a truly lonely man he was and how lonely at the moment we all were. Unknowingly, we had seen the soul of this quiet loner, and so doing had glimpsed our own. The make-believe dog had become the man's only possession, an extension of both his real and his subconscious isolation, and in some ways, a companion he had always wanted.

The corpsman finally managed to snap Fred out of it, and we returned to our own tents in silence. Fred was left standing there, confused and half-smiling at the incident he couldn't really remember, and the candy-striped dog trotted off over the hill and into the warm summer evening. The incident became an element in the heart's memory of how close we are, dog and man. And how close we were, Barkley, Cinelli and me.

CHAPTER NINE

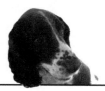

WE DID A LOT OF HIKING ON THIS TRIP, but we also did a lot more resting than we usually do. Most of it was to accommodate Bark, who was increasingly showing signs of weariness. When we'd stop, he'd not just sit but sprawl out flat, the way he'd done before his illness after a hard run in one of those leash-free parks. In some ways, we were in a state of denial, I guess, not wanting to believe that he was walking around with the fire inside of him, burning away his life. Cinelli would say "slow down" softly when she thought we were doing too much, and sometimes we'd sit a little longer on a park bench with Bark on the bench next to us, his chin on Cinelli's lap. He did this more frequently as the journey continued, almost as if he were seeking protection from that something inside of him that was sapping his strength.

One of the most difficult hikes was at the Newberry National Volcanic Monument south of Bend, Oregon, fifty thousand acres of lakes and lava fields. At the foot of eight-thousand-foot Mt. Newberry in the Cascade mountain chain, the lava flow stretched out like the terrain of another world, a gray and jagged landscape born in violence seven hundred thousand years ago and spewing ash and lava as recently as thirteen hundred years ago, when Mt. Newberry shrugged its mighty shoulders as a reminder of its potential. Experts warn, by the way, that it isn't extinct. They guarantee that it will blow again.

When you're meandering through the mountains, in no hurry, stopping a lot to look, to walk the dog and to be mesmerized by the beauty of the back roads, the rest of the world doesn't matter much. It's what this trip was all about in a way, to free us from the outside terrors that crawl through the long nights of unrest and violence, enflaming our world. We didn't watch television for almost the entire time and, uncharacteristically, I avoided buying newspapers, except for some community journals that couldn't care less about the rest of the world.

Our concentration was on Barkley. This was for him.

Mountains and oceans dwarf our human concerns, just as the immensity of cosmic space minimizes the features of our own small blue planet. For now, we're pretty much locked into a corner of the universe, albeit struggling to break free, and the size and grandeur of sea and mountains are what we possess to put us in our place. Only when hurricanes smash our cities, earthquakes tear down our monuments and volcanoes pour molten lava over the countryside do we realize how truly awesome these forces are.

Living on the West Coast, I've never been in a hurricane (and never want to be), but I have been through a few earthquakes. A temblor rocked our house one morning with no warning, even from Barkley. He looked up and around him when it happened then went back to sleep. This defied the theory of a self-proclaimed expert who appeared before a committee of the State Senate, claiming to possess evidence that dogs knew in advance when a ground shaker was coming and howled incessantly until it hit. Either Barkley, who was a puppy then, was not yet sensitive enough to detect the first quivers, or the man who offered the theory was less an expert than he thought he was. Bark hadn't made a sound before the 'quake. So much for dogs as seismic sentries.

Volcanoes are in a category by themselves, one of those awesome phenomena that combine just about every other form of nature's violence, including earthquakes, fire and the power to blow down anything in its way. Although not as huge as the historic eruption of Krakatoa in the Indian Ocean more than a century ago, Washington state's Mt. St. Helens gave us a contemporary lesson in vulcanology in 1980 when it blew its top. It was a reminder that, in addition to earthquake country, we live in volcano country. So naturally we had to see evidence of it.

One of the reasons we travel to the kinds of places others generally avoid for lack of fine restaurants or five-star hotels is because Cinelli, like Columbus and Vasco da Gama before her, is intrigued by the unknown and willing seek it out. Well, okay, we don't exactly sail uncharted seas or chop through the Matto Grosso (although we did struggle through a Panamanian rain forest once), but we do visit out-of-the-way locales on occasion and try to avoid tour buses like they were express transits to hell.

In quest of a volcano's fury, we passed on driving to the top of Mt. St. Helens because that's where everyone—I mean just *everyone*—goes, and Cinelli was, and still is, emotionally incapable of joining the mobs. That's how we ended up picking our way down pathways through fields of solidified lava at Mt. Newberry.

The intrigue of its potential is what lured Cinelli to a mile-long path through an obsidian flow, with Barkley and me trailing along. It was a fascinating but difficult trek, sharp rocks and an often narrow path making anything on the level of a casual stroll difficult. The dog expressed his interest by sniffing, barking and tugging gently at his leash, yearning for those days when his tugs could disconnect my arm from my shoulder. We were rewarded by his decision not to mark the perimeters of what he might consider his turf by urinating on the lava, having decided, I suppose, that it wasn't really his.

I don't think that nature's wonder was lost on Bark. He was absorbing the landscape, as we'd hoped he would. Every once in a while as the trail wound upward he would pause and stare out over the vast expanse of hardened lava. While one never knew if he actually understood the significance of what he was seeing, I have a feeling that in his little dog brain there was a sense of awe at its immensity. We are all in some ways little bits of eternity, and while our place in the grand design may be minimal, we are nonetheless a part of the greater universe that glows each day with life, both cosmic and molecular.

I don't mean to imply that Bark's illness was all a

downward spiral during our various hikes. While periods of weakness and weariness had become more common, he was also capable of explosions of energy. He could prance the full length of his adjustable leash and want more, while others, who walked dogs obediently at their heel, glanced at us to wonder why we didn't spend the time and effort to train our senseless beast. The Newberry hike, while nothing compared to what rock climbers undertake, would have been bad enough without Bark yanking at the leash, but we somehow managed it.

Heading south again, we weren't done with volcanoes yet. More lava beds lay ahead in California, just across the Oregon border, and just beyond that Mt. Lassen, the Golden State's own testy, eight-thousand-foot volcanic mountain that blew in 1914 and continued to sizzle for another six years. But first we had to deal with getting there.

I like to drive. I have no trouble zooming along on high-speed freeways or taking it easy on country roads, although I prefer the latter to the former. I can sit behind the wheel for hours without exhausting myself, stopping every once in awhile to stretch and walk the dog. When I do tire, Cinelli takes over and leads us safely to wherever we're going. Living in L.A., I've even managed to more or less accept its awesome traffic, if once in awhile I can seek roads of less madness and congestion. But something is happening to those quiet roads. The RVs, shudder, are changing them.

There are roughly nine million recreational vehicles on the road today in the U.S., and I have no doubt that most of them were in California during our Barkley Journey—in front of, behind and on each side of us. They ranged from vehicles the size of Greyhound buses to relatively tiny pop-up trailers. There were forty-foot-long fifth-wheeled trailers and slide-in campers situated on the beds of pickup trucks. Some towed cars, boats and off-road vehicles, often at the same time, and others were VWs hauling trailers larger than PT boats, swaying along behind them. They were like semis either lumbering up steep grades, piling traffic behind them, or hurtling down the highway like hot cars at the Indy 500.

I've had a little experience with slide-in campers on pickups and a small, self-contained RV, and I am not to be numbered among their fans. We crossed the U.S. in one camper and drove through Mexico in another, and in both cases I couldn't wait to get out of them and into a motel, even a bad one. The self-contained mini-motor home was a Chinook, and if you like living in a rolling submarine and being battered by winds that can easily sweep a high-sided vehicle off the road, a motor home may be for you. We bought the Chinook with the idea of saving money on our various journeys through the state, but eventually gave it up when I began refusing to sleep in a space roughly the size of a coffin.

Both the camper/pickup combinations were rented. One broke down in a Mexican desert, where friendly locals repaired it, and the other I put on its side during a sleet storm near Oklahoma City. No one was hurt, but we were forced to spend a week in nearby Enid where both our money and our enthusiasm for the open road temporarily ran out. That was the family trip that included Hoover the mutt, and getting him back into the camper after it was repaired was an exercise in patience and exertion. The accident terrified him. We had to carry him to the camper door and manually shove him in and slam the door fast to keep him there, whimpering all the way. We made it home in weather meant for penguins, and while the trip roughly paralleled one of *National Lampoon's* "family vacations," with many of its disastrous turns, I was happy to be alive.

Bark never seemed to be terrified of anything. He adjusted to it all, even when an occasional raccoon or coyote popped its head out of the underbrush. One had to surmise that his hunter instincts had been dulled either by his illness or by the ease of a domestic existence. Otherwise, I guess, he'd have been after them for dinner. On one hike a jackrabbit hopped across the trail in reach of the dog's teeth. The creature paused in surprise, exchanged glances with Bark and then hopped off.

"The fool is suicidal," a startled Cinelli said, as Bugs Bunny bounced away into the forest.

Maybe so, but it was a part of the experiences we had hoped for our gentle little Springer Spaniel, life telescoped into a few memorable weeks.

CHAPTER TEN

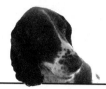

I SAW SNOW FOR THE FIRST TIME during the war in Korea. I emerged one morning from a squad tent and what had been mountains of darkness the night before, pocked with shell holes and burned by napalm, was now a glistening white. It had snowed during the night, silently, softly, cloaking with a mask of purity what the armies of contention had made so ugly. I remember staring in awe at the endless expanse of whiteness and understanding for the first time the stories of wonderland that I read as a child. I speak of it now because on the slopes of Mt. Lassen, it was Barkley's first view of snow, and his last.

We didn't dwell on it, even though acute lymphocytic

leukemia was something that just didn't go away. We understood the nature of the ticking clock, but chose to ignore the diminishment of time as we explored California's most recent volcanic mountain, and the fresh snow that was piled high in drifts along the upward road that encircled its 10,457-foot peak.

Barkley was transfixed by the brilliance of the scene, white snow gleaming under skies as blue as a starlet's eyes, the very air crackling with the effervescence of an arctic dawn. As we drove through it, looking for a place to stop, he stuck his head out the window so far I thought he might topple out. Had the window been open further, he probably would have. This was a new wonder in his life, just as it once had been in mine, and he wanted desperately to test it, to smell it, to touch it, to experience it, to absorb it. Nature has that kind of appeal, an allure that beckons like the song of sirens in the temptations of mythology. He didn't bark, he simply stared, pushing into the window's open space.

I had not expected snow. Cinelli, I learned later, had been told at the information center that it would be there, but kept it from me, realizing that my driving preferences cant toward a dry, open road on a sunny day. What lay ahead was a wet and often slick two-lane highway, one in each direction, that wound precipitously up over a mountain that suffered careless drivers poorly.

It was not our first trip to Lassen National Park. When our daughters, Linda and Cindy, were ages three and eight respectively, we had camped near Lake Manzanita, a bright blue body of snow-fed waters near the north entrance, in a campsite protected by a thick grove of red-barked manzanita bushes. They grow in tangles up to six feet in height, bunching at the top, but with enough room near their footings for, say, a child to crawl through. A child, perhaps, named Linda.

It is one of those incidents that remains in memory like the last traces of a nightmare. One minute she was in sight, playing with her dolls, and the next she had vanished into those secret places where babies, once they learn to walk, head for. Linda was, and still is, a born wanderer, inheriting from her mother a tendency to go someplace where she hasn't been. In this case, we had no idea at first how she could have disappeared so quickly. Cindy had always stayed close, more inclined to hang around than to drift off like a twig in a stream, but Linda . . . We knew of her tendency to wander, so how could we have allowed her to vanish on Mt. Lassen? It is a trick of the mind to go blank at critical intersections, thus allowing for dire consequences.

We weren't far from the lake, which was our first concern. Linda loved the water and would someday become a powerful swimmer, but at the moment, she was a toddler and nowhere near being able to conquer the cold water of a mountain lake. We had a dog with us, because we seem to always have a dog with us. His name was Grizzly. He was probably the most annoying pet we've ever had, absolutely untrainable and unresponsive to command or suggestion, with the possible exception of a "Come here" that involved food. Even then it wasn't a rush to his bowl, but a suspicious, and possibly arrogant, saunter in food's direction. Barkley he wasn't.

Any suggestion that we unleash him to find Linda was, on the face of it, ridiculous, since we had discovered during Grizzly's lifetime that he could barely find his way home, often wandering for miles until someone who recognized him dragged him into their car and brought him back to us. More often than not, his favorite place was the middle of the street in front of our house, which was then in the hills of Berkeley. Drivers of cars blocked by his presence could honk their brains out but Grizz wouldn't move until the driver got out of his car and chased him away, often employing language that would make a sailor blush, such was the degree of frustration the dog could cause.

But by the time the driver got back into his car, Grizzly was in the middle of the street again, testing the threshold of violence that kept the driver from beating him with a tire iron and discarding his body on our porch. Unleashing him to search for Linda was like relying on a mouse to search out a cat. On a scale of one to ten, Barkley being a ten, Grizzly was in the minus category. So we left him tied up at the campsite and set out with Cindy in tow to find Linda.

After about fifteen minutes of frantic searching and of accusing each other of failing to protect our young, Cinelli and I both heard a faint child's voice. It came from the center of the manzanita grove. More conversational than panicky, we knew instinctively that Linda was just having a good time in there, not calling to us but talking to herself, which she did for years into her childhood. I did the same as a kid, creating a character called Bob McCoy, with whom I had several conversations and a few hard disagreements. I still have fantasy visions. I think most writers do. It's the Walter Mitty Syndrome, the creation of whole new existences in your head. "Sometimes," Cinelli said to me once, "I don't think you live your own life." Maybe not.

We had to fight our way through the manzanitas to retrieve Linda, like natives hacking through a rain forest, scratched and bleeding from sharp branches, but we got her out all right. We thought about buying her a leash but that seemed so dog-like and possibly against a child-protection law, that instead we just doubled our watch, so to speak, and never let her out of our sight.

We visited that same campground with Barkley, or at least what we thought to be the same campground. Nature never remains constant, growing and shifting as the seasons blow by, altering the landscape that had once seemed so familiar. It changes the Earth as it changes our bodies, aging our faces, loosening our muscles and adding lines like roadmaps of a long journey to our faces. Men and mountains grow and diminish in the relentlessness of time.

Barkley sniffed around and barked once or twice at the animal smells that rode the winds circling down from the summit and through the fir and pine trees that pointed like needles toward a buttermilk sky. Among the vast differences between Barkley and Grizzly was that Bark responded. When you fed him, he ate, when you petted him, he wagged his tail, when you called him, he came. All of these traits allowed us to free him now and again even in parks that required leashes, knowing he would return instantly when we called him, should a ranger suddenly appear. Breaking the law is not what I usually do. I don't rob banks or mug old ladies (or even young ladies), but there seemed no harm in allowing a very ill dog to have the pleasure of a short run occasionally. How often would he be able to do this, to experience, unfettered, the freedom of California's high country?

What brought us there in first place was the peak's status in the Cascades, a mountain chain that includes St. Helens, a sister in the ring of fire that circles the Pacific rim and periodically shoots flames and ash into the unsuspecting air. Lassen began roaring its link to a primeval past by suddenly and dramatically blowing its top almost a century ago. Forces that helped shape the Earth were unleashed in a wild display of fire and smoke, reminding us that the core of our planet was still alive and active. A plume of ash billowed seven miles into the atmosphere and covered houses, cars and fields two hundred miles away with the darkness of a witch's veil.

The eruptions continued for a year or so, altering the immediate landscape and leaving evidence of their violence. The blasts devastated a large area of the mountainside, blowing down trees with the ferocity of a super-storm and scorching the land with blowtorch heat. While nature continually restores what seems to be eternally destroyed, remnants of the mountain's past are still obvious in boiling mud pots, hot springs and steam rising from cracks in the terrain.

We encountered snow about forty-five minutes from the north gate of the 106,000-acre park. It was reminiscent of another trip Cinelli took me on, that time to Crater Lake, one of the snowiest places in the nation, when a storm blew in and visibility was so bad we couldn't even see the lake. We returned the following summer just so she could see Crater's sky-blue water and realized that one of the reasons we couldn't find it that first time was that we were looking in the wrong direction. I had insisted, as I often do, that it was that way when it was actually *that* way. But we couldn't have seen it anyhow.

At Lassen, snow began appearing in splotches of white along the road, and as we climbed, the drifts became thicker and higher until there was little doubt by its height and purity that it was new snow. It was melting down over the winding two-lane highway, making its switchbacks seem more challenging than they probably were.

Barkley couldn't have cared less about the conditions of the road. There was amazement in his eyes as he stared at an ever-expanding vista of iridescent white, up mountain slopes and in sheets that flattened out into complex patterns in the alpine meadows below. The views were more than breathtaking. They were hypnotizing. One can easily understand how a sameness of the land, whether desert sand or mountain snow, can mesmerize one into an almost somnambulant state. Water appears where dunes roll and distant horizons where clouds exist.

I, however, am nothing if not dedicated to safety, having learned in combat how lack of attention to one's role could end in disaster. It was not a big tourist time, so the presence of Space-Shuttle-sized motor homes in the high country was limited, but motorcyclists buzzed around us like flights of wasps, their drivers seemingly clueless about the dangers of a road that was becoming increasingly slick as it wound to its summit at 8,500 feet.

Bark was going crazy in the back seat, jumping from one window to the other, afraid he might miss an instant of the silvery landscape that stretched out on both sides of the highway.

"We'd better stop before he crashes through the back window," Cinelli said. Indeed, he was that frantic. The decision to pull off the road came at just the right time. We rounded a curve and there was a small settlement that included a parking lot, bathrooms and cracks in the mountain where steam hissed into the frigid air. It was called, appropriately, the Little Hot Springs area, with a bridge that crossed to an area where one could be in reasonably close proximity to the actual hot springs.

A strong smell of sulfur in the air was no detriment to Barkley's joy of at last being freed from the confines of the car and leaping into the snow of this new and alabaster world. I kept him on a leash at first as he explored the terrain, pushing his nose into it, licking it and studying it up close for the first time. His paws sunk deep into a drift, which puzzled him at first, but not for long. The question of why his feet would sink into this white ground was simply a reason to do it over and over, and shake each paw free of the snow as it emerged.

"I wonder if there are snowshoes for dogs," I said, watching Barkley plunge through the snow in galloping leaps. It was one of those times when all signs of illness evaporated, overcome by an electrifying new experience. He stayed pretty much on the edges of the deeper drifts, eliminating the danger of sinking completely out of sight. It was as much fun sharing his exhilaration as it was being there ourselves. To see new elements of nature up close is to be absorbed by them. Going overseas aboard a troop ship in 1951, we were hit by a typhoon in the Sea of Japan, and I can still hear the roar of the storm and feel the sting of the ocean crashing over the deck. There will likely never come another time when I will be so embraced by wild weather as I was then.

While Bark's experience in tasting the first snows of his life couldn't really compare with the ferocity of a typhoon, it was as much a first for him as the ocean's violence had been for me. I went on from there to other experiences, but I knew as I watched Barkley test the new, white earth of his existence, that the limiting nature of his disease was building barriers around the days that remained for him. After romps through the snow, he pretty much collapsed on the back seat. I'm not sure if exhaustion was a result of the disease or of the strenuous activity. Maybe both.

That night, just outside the south gate of Lassen National Park, we stayed at what appeared to be the only motel in the minuscule town of Mineral, population 143. It was a cluster of buildings surrounding a restaurant and the motel office, which was a part of a store. The desk clerk, who also ran the store and probably owned the whole place, was a laconic, craggy-faced man with a sour demeanor whose manner indicated that he probably preferred to be left alone. He was reminiscent in appearance of actor Hugh Laurie, who played the wry and snappish Dr. Gregory House on the television series *House*, but lacked the script-provided wit.

He proved to be a totally humorless man and probably one who adhered to strict company rules, so I didn't tell him we had a dog with us, in the event that it was a place that didn't allow animals, and then where would we go? I actually couldn't see why we would be forbidden to bring in a dog or an otter or a dozen fat pigs, since the room was hardly in first-class condition. Well, yes, it would have been too small for a herd of swine, since a bed and a dresser ate up most of the space. The sink was also in the sleeping quarters, and the bathroom left barely enough room to turn around, even if you were, well, sitting, a situation that proved almost as intolerable as it was uncomfortable.

However, it was late, we were tired and I wasn't about to try searching out another motel, so we snuck Bark into the room. We ate at the motel restaurant that night and ordered a separate steak for the dog, whose presence, of course, we didn't mention to the waitress either, leaving her to believe we planned on a late-night snack of a cold T-bone. I tipped her nicely and explained nothing.

Barkley had no problem settling down on the floor near our feet. I see him clearly even today, caught in a diagonal of moonlight streaming in through a crack in the louvers, content to be with us wherever we were, that darling little dog proving even into his last days that he was one of us. The moment still shines in my memory.

CHAPTER ELEVEN

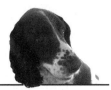

SHARMY WAS NOT A DOG ONE PALLED AROUND WITH. Grumpy and standoffish, he would snap when touched in the wrong places, but we never knew which places were the right places. We kept him away from small children, although he never really bit anyone. His snap was more a gesture of annoyance than attack. It was the wolf in him, I guess, that caused him to suffer with reluctance most contact with the human race. He was best left to ponder alone his place in our family, running with a pack in the open forests of his dreams.

He was our son Marty's dog, sharing the household with Lisa, Nicole and Jeffrey, wife and kids in that order. A third child, Joshua, was born after Sharmy had come to live at our house, and it was probably just as well. Unlike his siblings, Josh would not have treated the dog with respect, but probably would have insisted he ride him around the house, thereby coming into confrontation with the animal's uneven nature.

Marty asked if he could leave Sharmy with us while he built a fenced yard to contain him. Even though they lived in a five-hundred-acre wilderness park owned by the conservation district Mart worked for, Sharmy was not one to be let loose. Given his wolf genes, he would have probably ended up feasting on the small animals in the oak forest that surrounded their home or being eaten himself by a pack of coyotes or maybe even a mountain lion, whose screech one heard occasionally in the mountain fastness.

Since our yard was fenced and since Barkley might enjoy the company, we said yes. But what was supposed to have lasted a few weeks or maybe a few months, turned into an eternal residency. But for all of his cantankerous nature, Sharmy and Barkley seemed to adjust after awhile, establishing a kind of détente that humans might emulate. They never really fought, although there was an occasional lunge by Sharmy in Bark's direction when the latter became too much of a nuisance to the former. When you stop to think about it, it would be damned annoying to have someone nipping at your behind all day and jumping on you when you least expected it.

I mention Sharmy at this juncture because it was during this segment of the Barkley trip that our son, who was watching our house and taking care of the dog, our fish and our two cats, informed us that something was wrong with Sharmy. It was those words, offered in a similar context, which first alerted us to Barkley's illness when my wife and I were traveling in Wales, and now they were coming at us again. We were in Susanville, a town of seventeen thousand souls on the eastern edge of California, snuggled in the foothills of the Sierras at an elevation of about four thousand feet.

"I noticed he seemed to be bumping into things so I took him to the vet," Marty said. "She said he was going blind."

A genetic disease called progressive rod-cone degeneration had hit him with startling suddenness, turning his world first a faint gray and then totally dark. Scientists believe it is the animal form of retinitis pigmentosa, a leading cause of human blindness. We knew Sharmy was reaching a point of old age, but since we never quite knew how old he was, his exact age was uncertain. Even blind, he seemed to instinctively know his way around, although his pace had slowed considerably to a level of caution. He could move into the fenced yard through the dog door, and then into his special house, and he could find his own food and water (and, when we returned, Barkley's food too), but the perimeters of his life had definitely shrunk.

He snuck out of the house once when the front door was accidentally left open, and was found wandering in a gully not far away, unable to find his way back home. A neighbor spotted him bumping around in unfamiliar territory, obviously not knowing where he was, read the phone number on his collar and called our house. Sharmy was returned wiser for his misadventure, but otherwise none the worse for it.

Cinelli and I have owned many dogs over the length of our fifty-five-year marriage. We know that they can die for a variety of reasons, the best of which is old age. Grizzly, Hoover, Blue, Barney and Pooh all died in their senior years and of natural causes. Barkley was the first pet we had to die of an actual disease, and Sharmy the only one to go blind. The saddest of ends was met by Squirt, who was struck and killed by a car at Lake Isabella, north of L.A. Until then, we had visited the lake often. After that, we never returned.

Death is often sudden, a visitor who enters without knocking and claims its victims not by accident, but by natural causes in old age. My father died of a heart attack at age eighty, one moment alive and vital, and the next gone. Joan Didion wrote in her book *The Year of Magical Thinking* about the sudden death of her husband, John Gregory Dunne, while they were preparing for dinner: "Life changes fast. Life changes in the instant. You sit down to dinner and life as you know it ends." Because my parents were divorced, I rarely saw my father until after I returned from the Korean War. And then he was an integral part of my life and the lives of his newly discovered grandchildren. When he died, there was emptiness in my life, a horrendous realization that he was no longer there.

"Life changes fast. Life changes in the instant . . . "

My mother's death was equally sudden, of a stroke at age seventy-six, drifting off into the secret darkness of her body's confinement, her last words in Spanish, a language she hadn't spoken since she was a child, and could barely remember as an adult. One moment vital, one moment taking old-lady buses to gamble in Reno, one moment having her hair done for lunch with the girls, and the next moment, a memory.

Dying is a journey we take alone, but it can be a gentle departure, without pain or trauma, and without the agonizing notion that a life was ending too young and unfulfilled. At age seventy-six, I think about it occasionally, wondering what that final journey would be like, curious but not fearful of nature's course, trying to believe that Barkley's way would be no more than falling easily into his dreams.

Not intending to dwell on the morose, an impending sense of death was more on my mind in Susanville than elsewhere at the moment, because it represented the start of our journey home. Los Angeles lay approximately six hundred miles south and there would be other stops along the way, but the final destination wasn't some quiet mountain village with a single motel and a steak house. It was a sprawling, freeway-locked, multi-million-population megalopolis where life would involve more calamitous priorities, and for all it had to offer, L.A. is not a peaceful place. Gone is the kooky, laid-back image it once possessed. In its place is that of an emerging giant, howling its dominance for the world to hear, a monolithic, kinetic, muscular presence on the Pacific Rim of the world.

Contrarily, Susanville, barely larger than a village, was the perfect essence of a small town, with basic amenities available, but not on every corner. One felt oddly at home there, as though it had been part of another life, which, though it sounds a little spooky, created a familiarity that couldn't be denied. By the manner in which Bark quickly acclimatized to it, one would assume he was also taken with a sense of belonging.

My prior trip to Susanville had been as a reporter covering a civic uproar resulting from a theater owner's attempt to show an X-rated movie, *Behind the Green Door*. The police chief, mayor and a God-fearing Episcopalian pastor had demanded that the film not only be withheld, but be burned, torn up, stomped upon and otherwise destroyed beyond future use. They were not timid in their condemnation of smut. That was in the early 1970s, long before scenes of frontal nudity and writhing sexual encounters had become almost commonplace. The theater owner stood on his First Amendment rights for about fifteen minutes, then buckled under a purist onslaught. *Green Door* was never shown.

Our motel, only a few blocks from the theater, was a chalet gone to seed, but in the piecemeal stages of remodeling. Its attendants were two women of totally opposite character, one large and masculine, the other whispery and as skinny as a chopstick. Told we had a dog, the big one shrugged and the skinny one, lounging on a porch just outside the back door of the motel office, said, "I love dogs," in a voice so toneless that whether or not she loved dogs remained as much a mystery then as it was before she spoke.

We couldn't get into our room. Try as we might, the key wouldn't turn and the door wouldn't open. A handyman almost as thin as the office attendant came to assist. A cigarette never left his mouth during the twenty minutes he worked on our door, kicking it once or twice when his more productive efforts to correct the defect didn't work. He muttered unintelligible words around the cigarette and winced against the smoke trailing upward into his eyes.

All this time Barkley sat before the front door looking eagerly straight ahead, anxious to get inside and explore another interior world. His expressions were so clear that we never for an instant doubted what was on his mind. He was endlessly curious about what lay ahead, whether it was in the next city or the next room. His mouth hung open as he panted with excitement and his eyes burned with anticipation. As his frustration grew, his tail thumped on the porch in front of the room, reflecting our own impatience as we waited for the smoker to complete his work.

"Patience," Cinelli whispered to Bark, and he glanced at her as if to indicate that patience was for those with no place to go. He had a destination, which was inside of our room. His tail thumping grew louder and a low grumble sounded from deep within his throat. It wasn't a growl exactly, because he rarely growled, but a verbal indication of his need to get on with things. Given voice, he'd have probably said, "Can we go in now?"

The repairman finally replaced the entire entry hardware, knob and all, allowing us into a room that seemed similarly unfinished, with a door that still took all of our strength to open and close. The motel was my choice because its chalet shape reminded me of a place on northern Italy's Lake Como, but any similarity ended as we entered the room. To say that it was unfinished belies its state of dishabille. Holes in the wall remained where heaters had been removed, another where a light fixture had once been installed. It was as though the room had been abandoned in mid-remodeling, even to the extent that it lacked light globes in the remaining fixtures. Had it been looted of its heaters and its light globes, one wondered? The bathroom door, like the front door, took the full strength of both Cinelli and me to open and close, and even then it never did shut completely. We were just as glad, because being trapped and dying in a bathroom by a door that wouldn't open wasn't our idea of a perfect afterlife.

We didn't set up Bark's cage, because no matter what he might have done in the room, it would not have adversely affected its, well, ambience. He enjoyed the freedom, poking around into the corners of the unit, and then sprawling on the soiled carpet whenever he decided it was time for a nap.

Dinner was at a restaurant/jock bar called Champions. We were told it was the best eatery in town, and in fact it seemed to be the only eatery in town, other than the rows of fast-food places that lined Main Street. By now, Bark had become used to waiting for us in the car, knowing that something delectable would be forthcoming from our visits to good-smelling places. So he would alternate between sticking his nose out an opening in the rear windows and barking at passers-by or sprawling comfortably on the back seat.

As it turned out, Champions wasn't a bad place to eat, except for a martini drenched in vermouth. The modern martini, as prepared in places like L.A., San Francisco or New York, contains barely a whiff of vermouth. An example of that is a friend who simply waves the bottle over the top of his martini and whispers, "Vermouth." Our waitress was, judging from her dress, primarily a cocktail waitress. A woman in her middle years, she wore a miniskirt so short that it could have been a sash meant for her waist and never intended to cover any of her lower parts.

I saw pork chops on the menu and ordered some for Barkley, but was informed that they'd only had six that day and all of them had been ordered. "They got the last ones," she said, gesturing toward a couple more involved with each other than with dinner. They were in love, one would imagine, or at least sexually aroused, since they couldn't take their eyes or their hands off of each other. After the waitress had left us to mull over the rest of the menu and sip my bad martini, I wondered aloud if Cinelli thought it would be appropriate to ask the passionate couple if, due to the fact they were otherwise engaged, they would give up their pork chops, or at least trade them for something else.

"If you just went over and took them," she suggested, "they probably wouldn't even notice."

"Good idea," I said, rising from my chair.

"Don't you dare! I was only making a joke!"

"But I think you're right. Remember when we were . . . "

"Just sit down and leave other people's pork chops alone."

Lacking pork chops, Bark had chopped beef that night and didn't seem to mind a bit. He even devoured the mashed potatoes that came with his entrée, but not the broccoli, which he never ate. So I ate the broccoli, Barkley the 'burger. You might say we dined together. I was on a severe post-surgery diet once, eating nothing with any taste to it, while Bark was chowing down on a chunky dog food soaked with gravy. It looked a lot better than what I was eating and for a fleeting moment, I was considering a trade.

We took a walk after dinner at Champions, through starry nights and cricket sounds. The great outdoors are never far away in a place like Susanville. The creatures of the high Sierra dwell in the shadows. But living in Topanga Canyon, we're comfortable with whatever might be sniffing about in the foothills. The Santa Monica Mountains harbors all kinds of creatures, from coyotes to movie producers. Occasionally one hears the scream-like call of a mountain lion beyond the shadows. In other parts of Southern California there have been vicious attacks, but never in our canyon.

Rattlesnakes are equally at home among the artists, writers, conservationists and unreconstituted hippies who live among us. I have dispatched a few (rattlers, not hippies) with a shovel in our yard. Meeting one on a trail, I would let it live, but not where my grandchildren play or my wife tends her large and awesome garden. Some will bag the snakes and transport them to far-away places in the mountains, but I remember too well the lesson of a neighbor who tried that and was rewarded with a bite. Allergic to the anti-venom serum, he spent eight days in intensive care. A similar experience befell a woman who was bitten on the eye by a black widow spider that crawled on her during the night. Also allergic, she suffered the pains of hell before recovering.

But, still, walking through nature, or even near it, engenders a feeling of peace that one can never experience in a large city. Barkley sensed that occasionally and slowed to a casual walk, allowing one's right arm—the leash arm—to rejoin its socket. Cinelli and I walked him together after dinner, and we both understood that we were a trio that soon would be a duo. The evening was balmy, given over to the sweetness of a soft breeze that carried the faint perfume of pine trees into the foothills.

"He's comfortable with all of this," Cinelli said as she watched him sniff the ground and occasionally the air, wondering what was out there, or perhaps knowing what was out there, but not troubled by it. We walked him on the roads off Main Street, toward the surrounding forest. "I think he knows that there's something elemental to this trip."

"Yes," I said. "I think so."

We are an emotional but sensible couple who keep our passions under control most of the time. We can argue with the heat of Clarence Darrow and William Jennings Bryan debating the Bible for as little reason as whose turn it is to feed the dog, but on the larger issues of politics and morality, we are one; neither of us needs a chapel to reinforce our ethical standards. They remain firm without kneeling.

"He seems to reflect our moods. Maybe even our knowledge," I said.

"There may be more to the sensitivities of living creatures than we realize," she said.

"He misses us when we're gone," I said.

"Yes." Pause. "And we'll miss him when he's gone."

I kept thinking about it as the walk ended and we snuggled down under the covers, Bark at the foot of the bed. I sat up once to check on him, and, sensing movement, he looked up. Our gazes met. And I realized in that instant in the wee hours that he knew.

CHAPTER TWELVE

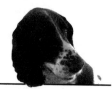

WE SWUNG WESTWARD OUT OF SUSANVILLE, stretching out the journey, fearing its conclusion, poking through the alpine passes, absorbed by the vistas. We played CDs to distance ourselves from the inevitable, John Denver singing mountain songs, along with odes to West Virginia, and to the sunshine on his shoulder. You get pretty much talked out when you're together on motor trips through days or weeks of sitting next to each other. You can't think of anything else to say. So we drove in silence a lot of the time, each in a separate world of spaces and daydreams, rummaging through our memories.

I realize that it might sound cynical to non-writers, like

the ultimate exploitation of someone dear, but I couldn't help wondering what kind of column I would come up with when leukemia finally claimed Barkley. There was no cruelty in my musing, no wish for him to die for the sake of a thousand words. I grapple with grief as I grapple with joy, examining both with a writer's curiosity. They become the same in the embrace of ideas. It's a thought process always running through the head of someone who creates.

I have often speculated with equal inquisition whether I would have time to write my own last column, or whether death would slam me down where I sat or as I walked, one minute alive, the next gone, as it did my father and John Gregory Dunne and so many others I've known over the years. I keep thinking that maybe I ought to write a last column now, but I'm simply not prepared to do that, for a lot of reasons, the main one being that I'm still not ready to depart, if you know what I mean. I cannot forget the anguished words of a good friend in his sixties, terminally ill with brain cancer. I was trying to help him through his last weeks and I thought he was accepting my solace until he looked at me and said in an anguished tone, "But I'm not ready to die."

One would like to think, but I am too much the realist to believe, that at some point there is a regeneration of life in a distant paradise, and that we will all come together, friends and old enemies, in an atmosphere of good will, free of old ailments and enmities, where music plays, where we dance and where gasoline is only twenty-five cents a gallon. We cling to the words of "ghost whisperers" who claim to connect bereaved survivors to their dead loved ones, profiting from their deep distress, and even achieving a modest level of fame, thanks to television's insatiable appetite for audiences. I talked to one of them once, James Van Praagh, the spiritualist's spiritualist, who was all the rage for a while. One's inclination is to dismiss people like him as frauds, but how do you prove he doesn't talk to the dead? How do you prove an itinerant evangelist preaching out of a tent *doesn't* talk to God? I asked Van Praagh if, as proof of his metaphysical talents, he could contact my dead dog Hoover and determine whether or not he is still in everyone's way. He replied somewhat testily that he could, but he was too busy and didn't like my attitude.

I wondered as we drove how I would handle Barkley's death, in professionalism or in pain, recalling with humor or tears his short romp through life? I didn't ask Cinelli what thoughts might be drifting through her head, although I could sense by her frequent glances at Bark that she too was thinking of the dog that lay stretched out in the back seat, considering his dreams.

It was an especially quiet time driving through the woods of Plumas County down a road with very little traffic, when Cinelli broke the silence by suddenly shouting, "Stop!" This kind of abrupt blast projects me into an immediate sense of peril not unlike a warning to "duck!" an unknown object hurtling toward me. Have I run over a farmer? Is there an asteroid heading our way? Has Barkley leaped out the window? I hit the brakes.

"What?" I demanded, on the edge of panic.

"Back there."

"Back there what?"

"That little restaurant. Let's have lunch there. It's quaint."

I guess, after a half-century of marriage, I shouldn't be surprised at her flashes of instinct that pick out a restaurant or a motel or a road more interesting, and usually better, than the average. This particular eatery was off on a side road she had spotted between the trees, a country place so typical it could have been built for a movie set. Even the people were typical, obviously plucked out of a group of Hollywood extras due to their ability to fit into a country setting.

I can't remember the name of the place or even exactly where we were, except that it was on a road that went basically nowhere. It could have been in Nebraska or on a potato farm in Idaho. I'll call it Mom's Place. I noticed as we peeked in the screen door that a couple of people had dogs lying next to their tables. I think it's illegal to bring animals into an eatery unless they're guide dogs, which these dogs obviously weren't. There were three of them in the restaurant, and all were large, hairy old animals of unknown pedigree. They slept as though they belonged there, indicating that this was an establishment where, as in Paris, you brought your dog, although Mom's was about as different from a bistro in Paree as Arnold Schwarzenegger from Jacques Chirac.

The restaurant was a wood frame building with a front overhang that shaded a porch with chairs on it. I was disappointed that the scene lacked old men chewing tobacco, watching the world go by and dejuicing themselves of the tobacco into spittoons at their feet, keeping count of who spat directly into the pots and who missed and spattered their juice on the floor. The chairs weren't only empty but they looked as though you'd go right through them to the floor if you did try sitting on them, such was the state of their disrepair.

We took Barkley in with us and were instantly confronted by a waitress the size of a Pittsburgh Steeler who

asked if we wanted blueberry pie. We had given no indication that we wanted pie, but it seemed prudent to say we'd
have some for dessert and then ordered ham and eggs, the
most prominent entrée on the menu. A Zagat-listed restaurant it was not.

"I'll bet they have good ham and eggs in this part of the
world," Cinelli whispered. "Their own chickens and their own
hogs."

"They must have their own blueberry fields too," I
whispered back, "because everyone in the place seems to be
eating blueberry pie."

"I'll bet Mom made it."

Barkley seemed pretty amazed by the fact that he was
in the kind of establishment where we usually went without
him and from which we brought back food. Under normal circumstances he'd have been all over the place, introducing himself to the other dogs, sniffing what was on the other tables and
generally being a pleasant nuisance. But this time, stunned by
his new acceptance in an eating salon, he just sat there looking
around, and kept looking around even while he ate the hamburger we'd ordered him. The ham and eggs were fine and the
blueberry pie wasn't half bad. Mom, or whoever the large waitress was, only charged half-price for the hamburger, deciding

that Bark seemed to be of the age where he could eat off the children's menu. I guess old dogs paid full fare.

As we drove off, Cinelli looked back and said, "I don't believe that place is real. We'll come back again and it won't be here and no one will ever have heard of it, like on *The Twilight Zone*. Stop so I can get a picture just to prove it once existed."

"Someone was probably murdered there," I said, backing up, "and it's doomed never to disappear. The waitress and the men and the dogs and the blueberry pie have probably been there for hundreds of years and will be there for hundreds more, unchanged. Maybe a whole family of hog or chicken farmers was wiped out there, beaten to death by a crazed handyman who burst in with a blood-stained scythe and . . . "

"All right, enough already!" she said after taking a picture. "Just drive. We'll come back in a hundred years and check out your theory."

And if time is a circle and the gods can do magic, we'll bring Barkley with us again.

CHAPTER THIRTEEN

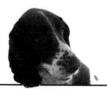

IT WAS RAINING HARD the afternoon we pulled into Yuba City, a small town north of Sacramento. It drummed against the car like a percussionist on steroids and blurred visibility to about a half a block. Water ran down the gutters and cascaded into storm drains with a force that blew spray into the gray air, and the high pitch of the wind was like a howl of pain—just as it had been in 1955 when the Feather River smashed through an earthen levee and left death and destruction in its muddy wake. Barkley had never seen a storm of this magnitude and spent part of the time twisting his head so he could look upward to the hovering origin of all this wind and water. I looked too, and my memories were as dark as the cloud-choked sky.

Among Bark's almost human traits was an ability to perceive change. I'm not saying he could forecast the weather by sensing a shift in the air pressure or anything like that, but he did seem to understand the difference in his surroundings. By staring at the sky it was like he was wondering why, when it was generally blue, was it suddenly dark in the middle of the day? At home, if we'd buy a new chair or add a different vase to a table he was right there sniffing and checking it out. Same with his journey. It was all different, and he was noticing the variations of the shifting scenes.

One of the good things about motor trips is the ability to veer off and visit friends. We picked off bits of my past with old buddies in Florence, Oregon, where they blew up the whale, and in Paradise, a town that retired L.A. Timesman Wil Locke regarded as sheer hell because of its marauding bears and dim-witted politicians. Yuba City presented an opportunity to visit a friend from my junior high school days. Jerry Kelly had lived in an upscale housing development during our teens in East Oakland. We occupied a ramshackle place nearby where we raised rabbits to sell as food for $1.50 each. It sustained us during the depths of the Great Depression.

Touching your past can bring back a lot of memories, not all of them good, some of them mixed. Like the Yuba City flood. It wiped out much of the town when the levee crumbled during weather almost like the kind we were experiencing on this visit, only worse. It happened on Christmas Eve 1955. It was one of those storms of the century that had been rolling over Northern California a good part of the month, and most of the state's rivers were already roaring out of the mountains like locomotives at full-throttle. The storm was accompanied by unseasonably warm weather in the high country, melting the snow pack and sending tons of additional water roaring down the Feather River, which divided Yuba City from Marysville, just on the other side.

Unable to withstand the pressure of a combined storm of the century and snow-water cascading out of the mountains, the levee broke at Shanghai Bend and sent a wall of water twelve feet high smashing through Yuba City, but sparing Marysville. Old-timers remember the sirens warning of the break and the thunder of the water smashing through homes and buildings, tossing cars in its wake, burying whole families in water and mud and debris. Power poles were snapped off and bodies left hanging on the branches of fruit trees in orchards that were laid out as far as the eye could see.

Death toll figures ranged from thirty-eight to seventy-two. Even those who keep track of these kinds of statistics still aren't certain. Damage was estimated at over twenty million dollars. I was a young reporter for the *Oakland Tribune* and arrived in Yuba City the day after the levee broke. I saw houses swept away by the power of the flood and deposited atop other houses. I saw cars hanging from power poles. I saw main thoroughfares still underwater. I saw helicopters plucking stranded people from rooftops and car tops. I saw stunned residents returning to a town that had almost ceased to exist.

It was different on this trip. The rain was letting up as we checked into a dog-friendly motel almost half a century later, but the skies were still as gray as a widow's eyes. Barkley greeted both rain and non-rain with equal enthusiasm. He could flop about in wet weather all day if given the opportunity, but I wasn't about to flop about in it with him, despite my own love of real winter weather, as opposed to eighty-degree Christmas seasons in L.A. While I don't mind driving in rain or even walking short distances in it, I prefer the warmth of a roaring fire while rain pitter-patters on the roof like the hesitant tapping of a stranger at the door. A sprinkle rather than a deluge. El Niño, stay home.

New levees have replaced the old ones at Shanghai

Bend, and new housing projects fill much of the flood plain swept clean of life by the 1955 break. We took Barkley for a walk atop the levee and then let him romp on the shores of the river. The sun had come out and there was sweetness to the air after the rain. The world seemed to glow in the dampness and in the water that dripped in a metronomic rhythm from the leaves of surrounding trees.

We picnicked by the river, and as I watched Barkley running and sniffing up and down its shoreline, I marveled at the resurgence of nature after a catastrophe. I noticed it revisiting Korea fifty years after the war. Trees had grown over mountains once scorched clean by napalm and shattered by heavy artillery. Time had filled craters blasted open by bombs, and covered them with chromatic arrays of wildflowers. Spring had reclaimed the land that men had tried to destroy. In the L.A. canyon where we live, raging brush fires had more than once blackened the chaparral into a surreal landscape of dark limbs that clawed like dead fingers toward the sky, and ash that lay like a thin, ghostly sheet of white over the dark hills. But time and nature spread life where they dance, and flowers follow.

In Yuba City, life had sprung into being again. Walnut trees grew in orchards once flattened by the unrelenting force of the water-storm that rushed through the break in the levee a half-century earlier. There was a lively bustle to business districts that had been inundated by floods, and a new sparkle to neighborhoods that once grieved.

It was a pleasant visit with Kelly and the girl, now his wife, he had loved since high school. Despite a friendship that covered depression and war, we remembered good times of growing up together and rushing through our teens with the speed of Olympians. They loved Barkley, who spent most of the evening in the car because he wanted to be too much a part of the dinner, demanding the kind of attention not offered at a party. You don't go to someone's home for a nice evening and bring your dog, unless you're either blind or a narc accompanied by an animal trained to sniff out crack cocaine.

There was an exception to this at a time when we owned two goats, Lucy and Melody, one a Saanen, the other a Nubian. Cinelli brought Melody inside during a dinner party we were hosting for other journalists after one of them doubted that we were true animal lovers. When Melody sauntered in and tried to stick her nose into his baked lasagna, I thought he'd fall off his chair. He never doubted us again.

In Yuba City, after dinner with our friends, we walked Barkley through a grove of trees off of a quiet road. Our journey was ending. This was the last stop in Northern California. Tomorrow we would head south and maybe stop once more, but the mountains would be behind us, and so would a sense of freedom that characterizes their intimate, village-sized towns. Life assumes a more formal mode as one approaches Los Angeles. It is a different cultural biome that spreads out to the visitor who comes down over the Grapevine into a world that mixes a blend of high-speed freeways with down-home folks; king-sized entertainment parks with small-budget movies; big money with small dreams.

"It's almost over," Cinelli said as we walked Barkley through the grove of trees. We could hear the river's rush in the near distance.

"It had to end," I said. "All things end."

"Do you feel the sadness?"

"Yes."

"I think Barkley does too."

"I think so."

"One wonders why it all happened."

We left it to the river and a soft wind and the starry night to ponder.

CHAPTER FOURTEEN

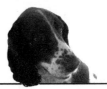

"I stood at a crossroads and fate came to meet me."

—Anonymous

JOURNEYS END. "Once upon a time" becomes the final pages of a story almost over. If it's a good story, one yearns for more, the way children cling to a glimmer of wakefulness before slipping into their dreams. But linger as we might over a tale well told, it must at some point conclude, at least in the original telling. What remains is the sweetness of memory that the narrative evokes, bits of images so precious that they become an integral part of us. Such is the story of Barkley.

We felt his life force fading even as we began the last lap home. We skirted Sacramento, past the gilt-domed capitol of California's ship of state, and began a day of driving on stiletto-like I-5, slipping past the sun-burned towns of San Joaquin County, slicing through fields of farms and orchards, down borders of hills and flat lands. Here was the heart of the Golden State, fruit and vegetable market to the world, its commerce rooted in the richness of the land and the unrelenting nutrients of the sun.

Barkley had held to his journey with the grace of a quiet hero, giving to us more than he gave to himself, draining the reserves of his strength to create the memory of a dog bouncing over new ground and sniffing new winds, filled with the excitement of discovery. If he seemed to sleep a little longer than usual or look at us in ways that evoked an inner pain, we chose to ignore those signs and revel in the pleasure of his company, of the nine years of joy and undemanding love he had given us.

It is approximately a six-hour drive from Sacramento to L.A., give or take stops along the way. It is a trip we have taken many times to visit our daughter Cindy in the capital city. It can be a quick trip if one is destination-minded, driving at high speeds down the strip of pavement that connects L.A.

to just about everything else in the state. But not this time. We chose the long way home in order to prolong this journey of the heart that would compress into a few weeks the life story of a very special pet. We savored the minutes the way one savors the lingering sunset of a special day.

To prolong the trip we veered over to Highway 99, the old north-south route to the City of Angels, a longer way home. Manteca, Modesto, Turlock and Merced slid easily from the foreground and into our rearview mirror, mingling with trucks piled high with fruit or hay, and the smaller vehicles of local commerce that buzzed like horseflies among the giants. Both I-5 and 99 comprise the lanes of transportation that link supplier with buyer, and they never sleep, not at midnight nor at four in the morning. Their drivers gather at the truck stops that feed them thick steaks and fries and coffee as black and thick as the La Brea Tar Pits.

We took our time, staying to the right, and finally veering westward on the kind of road that Cinelli loves, one that goes nowhere in particular. We were somewhere in Kings County, among the richest, flattest land that a farmer, or a food conglomerate, could hope for. It stretched all the way to a misty horizon in patterned squares of cultivation and ownership. Seen from the air it's a quilt laid over the earth, a pastiche in shades that blend and alternate, lending diversity to the landscape.

Barkley sat up when trucks thundered by on 99 and now was awake to the new scenes that passed. The mountains and towering pines were gone, replaced by strange vistas of flat-ness, and thin lines of waterways that irrigated the land. We stopped to let him inspect a land that had been transformed almost magically to the drowsing hum of the car engine. He greeted the newness with enthusiasm, but his legs refused to obey the desire of his soul. Running was hard, and even though he still tugged at his leash, it lacked the strength of the socket-jerking pulls he once managed. We walked slowly now, and let him absorb the smell that drifted up from the vast fields and inhale the distances that the fields comprised.

Back in the car, we wandered up this road and down that one, some without any names, bearing only the identifica-tion of a county number. No state highways cut through this terrain, but interconnecting lanes seemed to go everywhere and nowhere at once. Often lost, we stopped to ask directions, but stumbled on the language. Mostly Spanish was spoken here and, despite my surname, I can barely navigate through the ter-ritory of Hispanic words and idioms.

"It's that way," I said at one point, gesturing toward

a horizon.

"You determining a direction is like a cat cooking dinner," Cinelli said.

I admit I have a bit of trouble figuring out which way to go once we leave the driveway and it is occasionally, well, almost always, the wrong way. That's peculiar, because as a Marine in Korea I was ordered to teach map reading while in regimental reserve. The rationale was that a busy Marine was a happy Marine, even when resting, and since I'd had three years of college, I should be able to teach something, like the use of complex grid maps.

"No wonder the war lasted so long," Cinelli has often said. "You were determining direction and everyone was totally lost."

But this time was different.

"Look," I said, pointing, "the sun is in the east. An old Indian once told me that the east is always to the right, so that way must be north."

"Let's start from the beginning. It's two o'clock in the afternoon. So the sun is in the *west*, dear boy, and once more you would have had us traveling in exactly the opposite direction."

"Hmmm. So then that's east."

"Always has been."

As it turned out, that didn't do us a lot of good in getting back to Highway 99, where we had to be in order to continue south, which was, well, that way. So we just kept poking about with Bark sticking his nose out the window sniffing away, until we located the elusive highway, just as the lengthening afternoon was throwing shadows over the fertile land. The road home lay ahead.

We pulled into our driveway on an evening as warm and sweet as honey in tea. A full moon sailed through a breeze that laced our yard with the perfume of night-blooming jasmine. But the beauty of the moment was darkened by the realization of how far the disease had ravaged Barkley's body. I have watched close friends die of cancer, roaring out their lives almost to the end, when the body suddenly sags and the fight to live concludes with startling suddenness.

With Bark, the end came more slowly, over the next few months, with flashes of his old verve intermingled with moments drained of any animation. The oncologist said it would be this way, the disease exploding with the force of a thunderbolt, leaving pieces of life slowing disintegrating in the passing days.

During questionable times, we took Bark to our local veterinarian, who treated him with loving care, and he'd bounce back with vigor. That was before the disease that was probably locked in his system from birth burst out and into the open to claim its host. When, in Wales, we learned through our son's telephone call that Bark was truly ill, it was a red flag that would wave over his short future. The terrible prognosis that he would live for only nine months proved painfully accurate.

We watched him fade over the ensuing weeks through stages. Sue Downing treated him with a combination of life-sustaining chemicals, but the disease was winning. She cared for him with the warmth of a mother treating her son. We could see the differences in his response for maybe a day after treatment, but despite great advances in medical science, including those in the area of animal ailments, there comes a point when nothing more can be done. Refusing to accept ter-minality, we insisted that they try once more, something new, a miracle drug still in a laboratory's test phase—but the brain knows what the heart denies, that the end is near.

It had always been his habit at night when I'd say "Okay, Bark, bedtime" to bounce up the stairs with the eagerness of Tigger, the kinetic feline in *Winnie the Pooh*. As time passed, the response to my invitation became a slow, painful walk up the stairs, rather than a dash and a leap into the small, leather-covered couch that was his, and his alone. Then came the time that to navigate the stairs up to a mezzanine bathroom level and then to the bedroom level became an impossibility. First he would stop at the bathroom level, and, near the end, simply lie on the floor at the bottom of the stairs, looking upward, his eyes telling us of his defeat, and his sadness.

Toys that he once enjoyed, balls that lit up or squeaked, and puffy bears or bones or things that rolled, lay in corners or in the center of the living room, untouched, like the toys of a child who has gone away. Even as I write I can see them, sometimes tucked under a sofa with Barkley reaching for them with an extended paw, or down a hallway that ends at a guest bedroom.

On the last day of his life, I picked up each toy carefully and placed them in a wire basket where they were often stored, a gesture that seemed almost ritualistic in nature, like laying flowers on a casket. It was in the late afternoon on a day of oddly flattened light, when the world seemed very still and sounds muted. Bark's appetite had gone completely, and constant retching had left him debilitated. He lay on our tiled floor in a semi-coma. Sadly, we knew the time had come.

We drove in silence to the Beverly Hills office of his oncologist. As we suspected, there was nothing more she could do for him. One absorbs times of trauma with special attention to the surroundings, logging them in separate, isolated places in the soul, apart from passing memories. The treatment room seemed incredibly small and closing in, its pale walls suffocating and impenetrable barriers. I see Sue Downing with iconic clarity, her face a professional blank but her eyes filled with grief. I see Cinelli's expression, creased in pain. I feel the emptiness in the pit of my stomach.

Arrangements were made to take Barkley to a veterinary hospital not far away, where he was examined once more. There was no hope. The dog that had been Barkley had vanished inside the black-and-white animal with floppy ears that lay before us on a gurney. Downing's final opinion was affirmed. There was no life force, only pain. We didn't want a pet that had given us so much pleasure to suffer in the last moments of a life that couldn't be extended. I would ask the same for myself.

We knelt beside him, hugged him and said our last goodbyes. A flicker of recognition passed through his eyes, followed by a sadness that emerged from a place deep within. It was the last we saw of him. On the way home, we cried.

⁂

I'm not sure why the memory of Bark continues to tug like a magnet at my soul, but I keep applying it to so many events that he might have witnessed with us. It doesn't take a lot of concentration for me to visualize him slapping through the surf of Florence or barking at the smell of bears in Markleeville. I extrapolate from there to overlay his memories on trips we still take through the back roads of California, that wind into secret places by small streams, under an umbrella of pines or red-woods. We sit by a river eating a picnic lunch, feet dangling in the water, and suddenly an image of Bark splashes by, like a ghost from the forest, tail thumping against the surface, spray-ing us with water. I stare, I remember, and Cinelli, knowing, takes my hand.

A new animal addition to our family, a black cat named Ernie, fills in a little but also reminds us of Bark. Ernie, just a kitten really, tears at the paper that comes out of the fax machine the way Bark did when he was a puppy. And he stands, stretching, with forepaws on the dining room table to see what we're having for dinner, and would gladly take a bite if we'd let him. Just like Bark. Ernie talks endlessly, meowing a greeting at the door when we arrive after an absence, no matter how brief. Bark always met us there, happy to see us, sad to see us go. And at night, Ernie jumps on the bed for at least part of the night. Bark did that too, but always jumped off when it was time to sleep, and curled up on his couch.

We haven't replaced Bark yet with another dog. Truly, there is no way we could replace him. He was unique, and another dog would only suffer by comparison. We would expect him to understand that he could run freely up our driveway but stop at the street. Bark knew that. We would expect a range of emotions on his face that few other animals could manage the way Bark did. No rose is exactly alike, no sunset the duplicate of another. And no other dog could ever be our lovely Springer Spaniel. So we have Ernie the cat who, at this very moment, is sleeping on my desk next to my computer. He has many of the characteristics of Barkley, touching us with a paw, begging for attention, intent on playing, comfortable being near us. But he isn't Barkley, and never could be.

What else was it about Bark that made him special, different from any dog we had ever owned before? What spiritual inner force existed that connected him so remarkably to us?

What light shone? What compels me to write about him? I've thought about it many times, but there is no pre-packaged answer. Our relationship existed in deeper areas of our physiology, beyond the probing fingertips of our capabilities to adequately define it. Bonding is at the very least a combination of love, caring and a comfort in being near each other. We shared all of that with our happy Springer Spaniel.

As time passes, the pain of his death diminishes. While memory lingers, deep longings are soothed by the gentle passage of seasons. Barkley is gone from our lives, but not from our hearts. We look back with fondness at the years he gave us.

And we remember with love and gratitude that once upon a time . . .

IF ONCE YOU'VE HAD A DOG

By Jeffrey Martinez, Age 10

If once you've had a dog
You'll never be the same
You may look as you looked the day before
And go by the same old name.

You may have to chase her around,
You may have to pet her all day,
But you'll feel her nice, fuzzy fur
And hope she will always stay.

You may want to brush her a lot
You may want to touch her ears
Then you'll hear her loudly barking
And want to disappear.

Oh, you won't know why
And you can't say how
Such a change upon you came
But once you've had a dog
You'll never be the same.

ABOUT THE AUTHOR

AL MARTINEZ is a columnist for the *Los Angeles Times* and a native Californian. He has spent five decades covering the state and the nation for the *Times*, winning more than a dozen awards along the way. He was senior writer of a team that won a Gold Medal Pulitzer Prize in 1984 and a member of the Metro staff that shared Pulitzers in 1993 and 1995. Most recently he was honored with the President's Award of the Los Angeles Press Club. Martinez has written nine books and dozens of television screenplays. He, his wife, Joanne Cinelli, and their cat, Ernie, live in Topanga Canyon.

ANGEL CITY PRESS